TREATABLE
AND
BEATABLE

TREATABLE AND BEATABLE

Healing Cancer Without Surgery

CAROLYN GROSS

FOREWORD BY GERONIMO RUBIO, MD

Creative Living Publications
ESCONDIDO, CALIFORNIA

First printing 2007

ISBN 978-0-9718064-1-2
LCCN 2007920715

ATTENTION CORPORATIONS, UNIVERSITIES, COLLEGES,
AND PROFESSIONAL ORGANIZATIONS: Quantity discounts are available on bulk
purchases of this book for educational, gift purposes, or as premiums for increasing magazine
subscriptions or renewals. Special books or book excerpts can also be created to fit specific
needs. For information, please contact Creative Living Publications ,
306 NW El Norte Parkway #426, Escondido, CA 92026; ph 760-741-2762.

*To inspire cancer
patients and families to seek
the Treatable and Beatable mindset
in their healing journey from cancer.*

DESTINY

I don't recall the pain that brought me here
My how the joy takes the painful past away

'Tis a new season
Begins today
Grab a hold of now
And let your dreams unfold
Your Destiny is great
Your Story will be told.
—*Carolyn Gross, March 2000*

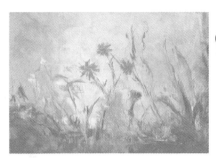

Contents

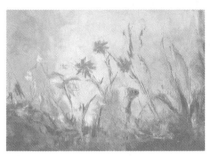

Acknowledgments

To my loving husband Bryan:
thank you for all your patience, strength, and assistance...
we only get better and better!

To the very special *Book Angel* for bringing me the talent team,
resources, support, and assistance on this special project, including:
Cheryl McPhilimy, Lorie Culp, Allan Burns, Starr Manson,
Aleta Pippin, Nancy Sielaff, Roberta Zito, and the
About Books, Inc. production and creative team.

Dr. Rubio and the entire staff at
American Metabolic Institute-Hospital San Martin...
thank you for saving my Life!

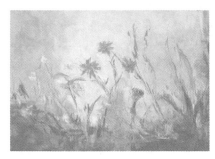

Foreword
by Geronimo Rubio, M.D.

This book is written by a patient of the American Metabolic Institute-Hospital San Martin to show the success of alternative treatment, combined with traditional methods, in healing cancer.

In recent years, cancer rates have risen to historic levels. A projected one in three Americans is now expected to develop the disease. It is an aggressive illness that requires an intelligent, aggressive response. My goal in treating patients has always been to deliver an in-depth treatment program customized for each patient, consisting of many protocols applied with flexibility and congruency.

The first time I met Carolyn Gross, I explained to her that cancer is a dramatic illness that demands a dramatic treatment protocol. The immune system of the cancer patient is typically burdened with other conditions in the body and is thus unable to deal with cancer. When cells grow and divide, they undergo a specific, regulated process called *mitosis*. Various factors such as viruses, chemicals, radiation, and genetics disrupt this process, causing abnormal cells to develop, grow, and divide uncontrollably. This is cancer.

Denial Is a Healthy Initial Reaction

Eight to ten years may pass before a patient begins to experience symptoms and a tumor finally appears. When symptoms arise, the tumor can exert pressure on the nervous system with resulting pain, or a large cancerous mass may be detected somewhere in the body. When most people are first diagnosed, their initial defense mechanism is denial, which is actually a healthy first response. In the days or weeks to come, patients must learn to deal with their illness on both psychological and physical levels. Several suggestions in this book will help people grasp these concepts.

Cancer cells are simple cells; they don't require a sophisticated scenario in order to multiply and become lethal. It is often thought that cancer results from a compromised immune system. However, even strong immune systems are unable to attack cancer cells because these wily invaders are encapsulated with a protein that prevents the immune system from recognizing and destroying them.

First Destroy the Coating— Then Destroy the Tumor

One of the first steps in dealing with cancer is to penetrate that encapsulated protein coating, which will then allow the cancer to be attacked. Tumor immunology is an integral therapy that I use as medical director at the American Metabolic Institute-Hospital San Martin. This cutting-edge treatment has been developed over the last twenty years, and our understanding of the immune system increases daily. As our knowledge grows, so does the potential to use immunological approaches as effective treatments.

Sometimes doctors, geneticists, biologists, and researchers forget that the human body is characterized by constant movement, that millions of metabolic reactions are taking place continuously; it is not a static situation at all. As the red cells, white cells, and blood plasma circulate through organs and tissues, the body cycles through different stages of energy. The immune system also undergoes millions of changes. It is imperative to train the immune system to recognize disorders and tumors and keep communicating these changes, so it can mobilize and destroy abnormalities.

I want to explain briefly how we can stop this cycle, arrest the tumor's growth, and maintain nutrition for normal cells at the same time, because cancer grows in an anaerobic cycle of fermentation. Cancer cells can grow without oxygen because they are anaerobic; they require specific nutrition and will steal all of the body's nutrients, thus depleting and stressing normal cells. They also produce specific enzymes that encourage new growth of veins and arteries, which attach to the tumor, making the tumor grow.

Various types of cancer are composed of many different kinds of cells; there are diverse causes and factors involved in over one hundred types of identifiable tumors. Many cancers are caused by food, environmental chemicals, and viruses—influential factors that we need to recognize and correct. Research also shows that some cancers are hormone-dependent.

Carolyn will discuss the nutritional approach we use as part of her treatment to successfully heal her stage three breast cancer. As part of the diet therapy I prescribe to my patients, I show them when and why a patient can endure a short period of fasting and how the prescribed diet will support immune system functioning. Then I work out a diet plan for each patient, according to blood type.

Addressing the Five Factors That Contribute to Cancer

The five correctable factors that contribute to cancer are: missing chromosomes, blocking factor, diet, hormones, and the immune system's inability to detect and destroy tumors.

Orthodox therapies such as radiation and chemotherapy used in conjunction with metabolic and immunotherapy contribute to our patients' successful treatment. In the healing environment at our medical institute, patients use revolutionary techniques such as *psychoneuroimmunology*, defined as the brain's ability to create cancer-fighting peptides through visualization. We also use a Rife frequency generator developed in the 1930s by a medical inventor to help destroy cancer cell bacteria and pathogens with an electronically transmitted frequency that matches the disease cells and deactivates them.

Someday I'd like to see the very term "cancer" eliminated from medical books, for most people react to the word with understandable fear. We need to replace it with a different terminology; perhaps we should refer to it as a "tumor disorder" or "immune B-Cell or T-Cell disorder," while explaining to the patient that her illness is unique and will be treated on an individual basis. Each of our bodies is composed of different genes and proteins, and we each have a unique ability to stop tumors from growing. With the right treatments, many patients can look forward to long-term recovery.

Even in the most serious cases, I encourage my colleagues not to tell patients how much time they have left. We're not gods; we're only human, and our mission as doctors is to save lives, not predict when our patients will die. We need to remember that the body can sometimes experience spontaneous remissions.

Through the use of customized, multi-faceted programs at American Metabolic Institute-Hospital San Martin, patients will respond better to traditional and complementary therapies. We feel that the patient is captain of his or her own body and needs to know when chemotherapy, radiation and other therapies will work and when they will not. If a patient has the desire and energy to fight the cancer, we can assist the body in rallying all its innate resources to win the battle.

For all the doctors, patients, and healers reading this book, it's time the world knows more about less invasive options to treat cancer successfully. At the end of this book, I give more specific information about the various vaccines I have developed over a twenty-year period. By reading about Carolyn's approach to claiming your power and gaining greater awareness, combined with the research we have done at American Metabolic Institute-Hospital San Martin, you will be introduced to an effective mindset and emotional approach to a cancer diagnosis, as well as the benefits of immunotherapy. These concepts and protocols are the most advanced therapies currently available. You will benefit from learning about how these remarkable treatments give patients new hope and a better quality of life.

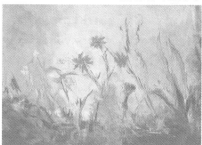

CHAPTER 1

Claiming
Your Power

I t was one of those days when I needed to remind myself that healing cancer without surgery is a huge undertaking. Fortunately, I happened to be at my hairdresser's, and Jacque offered me some much-appreciated support. Then she asked: "What I want to know when I read your book is how did you find the confidence to not have the traditional surgery and chemotherapy recommended by three doctors? Where did you find the *power* to do things differently?" I promised her I'd cover that in the book, and later realized this is the perfect place to start. When engaging in the battle with cancer, you need to claim your place of power the moment you are diagnosed.

Dry mouth, nausea, hair loss, surgical-removal of body parts, metallic mouth, fried taste buds, fatigue, depression, and an underlying sense of doom: this is the standard operating procedure for treating cancer in this country. Is this how twenty-first-century cancer treatment should be?

In the summer of 2003, I was diagnosed with stage three breast cancer. Always proactive with my healthcare and conscientious about annual mammograms, I found myself referred to a specialist who proposed the same treatment my grandmother had received thirty years ago—complete mastectomy, radiation, and chemotherapy. "And," the doctor added, "there are no guarantees."

A determined and informed consumer, I conducted research that led me to Mexico, where I met Dr. Geronimo Rubio, a physician whose successful treatment has helped hundreds. My results were remarkable as well. Within a year, the cancer was gone. I kept my breast and my hair and was spared the physical and psychological horrors breast cancer patients often suffer. Four years later, I'm a cancer-free woman—going strong.

Have You Ever Questioned Your Doctor?

When it comes to diseases and selecting treatment, our free will and power of choice are important factors that most people don't fully utilize. Many patients let doctors dictate how long they will live, how their lives will be changed, and even what they should believe. All too often patients are so shocked with the diagnosis and overwhelmed that they don't have the wherewithal to call time-out and do their homework.

I belong to a women's networking group, and I was certain that everyone there knew I had recovered from cancer without surgery. When Karen was diagnosed, I offered my phone number and said, "I've been there; if you have any questions about treatment, or anything, just give me a call."

Her doctors advised a mastectomy and two weeks later, Karen underwent surgery. She never inquired about my treatment, and I had to guess she assumed my doctors recommended no surgery. When I mentioned that I'd chosen immunotherapy, she had no questions to ask. I tried to extend her an olive branch of information or hope, but she never called. Not wanting to interfere, I waited.

Karen was in her sixties and stated before her surgery, "It's no big deal to lose my breast." But afterward, when she saw the scar, she had a change of heart. One day she wailed, "I decided too quickly. I *let them* talk me into surgery!"

My heart went out to her, making me more determined to inform recently diagnosed patients and their family members that they need to claim their power and investigate all options. You may well get some of your best treatment advice from other survivors, so use them as a resource. Inquire, search, and delve into books and websites like Adjuvant! for the latest research on how to treat cancer and support your body during treatment. Be open to help from others as well as to what's offered by your surgeon or oncologist. Bring your research to them, and see if you might be able to supply another piece of the puzzle. There is hope and there are options, and these pages will help you claim your power to find both. You have to believe in your healthcare team, treatment protocol, and yourself. Don't become a victim of your diagnosis; become a victor, and trust your instincts. It's these subtle nuances that are vital to listen to, even when you're emotionally reeling from the shock of diagnosis.

Before Karen's surgery, I'd once hinted: "Not everybody has surgery, you know." But she never asked, "What do you mean?" My offer went unheeded, so I knew all I could do was just observe her process. (For caregivers and loved ones, this is the reality.) It wasn't easy; there was so much I wanted to say, but I kept silent. Now I can share those unspoken words with you.

Your Body...Your Choice

I've talked to hundreds of women and men who want to surgically remove their cancer as soon as possible. This is understandable, since surgery has been the accepted treatment for years and years, engrained into us as the only way to solve the cancer problem. I've watched women diagnosed with breast cancer practically sleepwalk their way to the surgeon's table without a second thought. But it's important to wake up and find out what is right for you before you take a step like surgical removal of a body part.

You want to be confident and sure in your soul about both the treatment protocol and the doctors you select to have on your medical team. Don't cave in to hasty pressure. It took awhile for the tumor to develop, so taking a few weeks to get second and third opinions makes good sense and rarely puts one in jeopardy. I know there are exceptions to this rule with certain aggressive cancers, but you do have a little window of time for decision making. Use it!

According to the American Hospital Association, the number of hospitals offering Complementary and Alternative Medicine has grown from under ten percent in 1998 to nearly twenty percent in 2005. People have healed serious illnesses from these types of practices in conjunction with good medical treatment. After all, anything that relaxes the body heals the body.

I made my decision based on my study of the human body and my background in CranioSacral Therapy (an alternative health protocol that activates healing in the body). I'd learned through years of treating clients that so many things are possible when healing the body.

Collecting Evidence Theory

The *collecting evidence theory* means that as we journey through life and develop our particular point of view, we go out of our way to collect evidence to support those beliefs. In my case, I would consider surgery only as *a last resort*. As a result, I'm constantly encountering women who were traumatized by their hasty surgeries and their aftermaths.

I was on a routine visit to the hospital in Mexico for a vaccine when I met Vickie. As is typical in conversations with other patients, I asked, "What are you seeing Dr. Rubio for?" She replied, "Metastasized breast cancer." It was clear from looking at her that something wasn't functioning right. Her jawline was very swollen, both sides of her neck were inflamed, and even her shoulders looked like she had padding on them. I asked about her story. "I was diagnosed with stage two breast cancer," she said. "I was in such shock I just went along and did what the doctors dictated; after all, I did have cancer! I had a lumpectomy with four lymph nodes taken and then started chemotherapy. It was after the fourth course of chemotherapy I realized *this treatment isn't working for me.*"

This is actually the moment Vickie claimed her power. She continued, "The lumpectomy didn't solve anything; the cancer had spread to the lymph nodes, and it was then I began to do research on the Internet and through word of mouth. My research led me to a clinic in Santa Rosa, and when the doctor saw my advanced condition, he immediately referred me to Dr. Rubio for the cancer vaccine."

Vickie's case represents an important message. *Women and men need to claim their power the minute they are diagnosed, not after certain treatments are underway or completed.* In Vickie's case, when her cancer spread and she went back to the oncologist, he threw his hands in the air and said, "I can't help you."

A recent movie titled *Two Small Voices* quoted a statistic that caught my attention. It asserted that fifty percent of women have difficulty with implants after a mastectomy. Often these factors aren't considered when people are hasty or scared with their diagnosis and figure that the reconstruction surgery will make everything all right after they cut the cancer out.

Search and Research

In making a decision that will affect the rest of your life, do take responsibility for exploring every possible solution. Today with the Internet, it's easier than ever before. If you aren't computer savvy, ask a friend for help. Google (search for) your specific type of cancer or phrases like "cancer treatment," "alternative cancer treatment," or go to sites like Adjuvant! online. The Adjuvant! site, developed by Dr. Peter Ravdin at the University of Texas, provides information about breast, lung, and colon cancer treatments. Dr. Ravdin believes the patients who are active and informed participants are less stressed. There is also a Decision Board, developed by Dr. Timothy Whelan of McMaster University in Hamilton, Ontario, that helps doctors outline the treatment options to patients, so they better understand risks and benefits.

If the Internet isn't your cup of tea, visit the local library or bookstores and browse the books on cancer and health. Investigate those things that interest you; decipher and discern. Knowledge is power—there's a wealth of information out there, especially on the Internet—but it does come with a caveat. I caution you not to believe everything you read, especially on commercial sites or those with a self-serving agenda. In the Resource Section at the end of this book are some good websites for starters.

No matter what you choose to do, don't fail to get second or third (or more) opinions, and ask for referrals. Alternative clinics usually supply the names of former patients you can contact, and I believe traditional medical offices should do the same. Don't be afraid to ask your physician to put you in touch with three to five patients who have had a similar diagnosis and recommended treatment. At the end of this chapter are questions you can ask to help you in selecting your healthcare team and treatment protocols.

Taking the High Road

I happened to see Carly Simon on CNN with Paula Zahn, talking about her bout with breast cancer. Here was this talented singer-songwriter sharing the emotional ups and downs of her cancer journey. She said, "After cancer I have a broader range of emotional scales to write from."

She went on to state that her highs were now higher and her lows more intense. In a song on her CD *The Bedroom Tapes,* she expresses her way of dealing with her mastectomy, "I now have an arrow on my chest that points to my heart." Only an artist could describe a mastectomy scar in such poetic terms, and I applaud her.

Carly Simon also shared her initial reaction to her diagnosis. She had received the awful news over the phone, as I had. Her immediate reaction was to put the phone down, cry, and say, "This can't be happening to me!" I know how she felt, yet somehow I was calm, and like Joan of Arc on a quest, I knew early on I had to keep my wits about me because I had some important decisions to make. I needed to claim my power and explore my options.

It's also because of people like my friend Tom that I was able to keep my wits about me. Tom, who had been diagnosed with myeloma—bone marrow cancer—years earlier, is a very inspiring cancer patient.

He'd endured full courses of chemotherapy and was able to return to his professional speaker life. A few years later, as he so eloquently stated, *his remission was over.* This is what I call the "treatable and beatable mindset." Instead of saying *the cancer is back,* he declared, *the remission in temporarily over.*

When we talked further, he told me the next step his allopathic medical team had to offer was a bone marrow transplant. The treatment cost was $150,000, which meant that $25,000 to $30,000 was not covered by insurance. At the time we spoke, he admitted, in spite of his optimism, "I'm afraid this procedure will destroy my health even further."

I told him about my experience with immunotherapy and my belief that the answer to cancer treatment is in the blood. That day I gave him two phone numbers: one was the American Metabolic Institute-Hospital San Martin, offering Dr. Rubio's immunotherapy, and the other was Judith Reno, Ph.D. She is a five-year survivor of multiple myeloma, who underwent two bone marrow transplants to conquer her disease.

Because of Tom's investigative efforts, another option became available. He was selected to be part of a study involving a new treatment protocol. He was claiming his power: first, by giving himself the option to seek out other treatments when his gut warned him not to go with the bone marrow transplant and, second, by continuing to research other options. The study of the new protocol suited him—and it seems to be working just fine.

Finding Your Power in a Powerless Situation

As I mentioned earlier, my beautiful hairdresser challenged me to convey this concept of claiming your power, so people will be encouraged to participate in making their own decisions during a time like this. I want to offer you the following seven discernments as strategies to help activate this power, especially in times of crisis. For our purpose here, let's define discernment this way: to separate, divide, and distinguish between, to see or understand the difference, to discriminate.

These discernments embody the specific strategies I used to arrive at the choice to heal a 3.5 cm tumor in my left breast without surgery.

Discernment One: Listen To Your Body

Early on in my treatment selection process, I left the surgeon's office with his words ringing in my ears: "Nothing but a complete mastectomy." I drove home, took off my top, and stared at my breasts. There I was, forty-six years old, and my breasts were still attractive. When I attempted to visualize what I'd look like with one of them completely gone, my soul simply said, *it's not time to lose your breasts*. This revelation inspired me to keep investigating treatment options that were less radical, and it wasn't long before I found Dr. Rubio with his encouraging words, "Your prognosis looks very good."

We all get gut feelings. People will say, *I knew in my gut something was right or wasn't*. Or: *I listened to my gut and made my decision*. Your body has a lot to say, so in claiming your power, take the time to listen. The initial decision for me was very easy. It was later on down the road that I had my doubts and angst to conquer (more than a few times) about my treatment protocol.

Many practitioners in the healing arts see the body as an energy transmitter that receives messages from your soul and the external world. Your body will tell you when you are sick, fatigued, feverish, or if your blood pressure is up, just as it will tell you when you can feel safe or when you are being manipulated. Body consciousness in many ways is the true higher self.

A governing force in my life has always been my holistic approach to the body. I began to study nutrition at fifteen, believing that my body instinctively knows what is right, and I'm always looking for ways to encourage the body to heal itself. Years ago I made dietary changes that most people weren't yet considering. I eliminated sugar, wheat, and flour from my diet. This was before the low carbohydrate trend kicked in. All I knew was that when I consumed high carbohydrate foods I felt unhealthy, and when I eliminated them, I felt better. Because of my disciplines with food, I'm experienced at honoring my body by listening to its messages.

As a result of this philosophy and the dietary changes I made years ago, I don't over-indulge on weekends or at holidays and set myself back. These disciplines may not sound fun or delicious, but they offer a certain level of clarity. My body trusts me not to harm it, and my soul gives me accurate feedback on my surroundings, choices, and decisions. People used to ask me, in a slightly pitying tone, "Don't you miss chocolate? What do you do on holidays?" They were sure I was missing out.

As a cancer patient, sugar is not your friend. The bottom line is that sugar feeds cancer. I know that none of us is perfect when it comes to these types of disciplines, but we really have to toe the line when we are battling against cancer. This is especially true for people who are carbohydrate sensitive. Chapter Nine, The Self-Care Equation, will cover more on which sweeteners work for most people. Being a carbohydrate sensitive person, I don't indulge in any of the "'approved" sweeteners. This is how I keep things simple.

Because of these dietary disciplines, I've been listening to my body for so long that it's like any other art—you get better the more you practice. From these disciplines, I've become more attuned to the way my body sends me these signals from my spiritual center or soul, especially after having survived cancer.

I listen to my body when making decisions from the mundane to the life-altering. If a situation seems overwhelming when I merely think about it, the reality usually turns out to be the same. When I was first told, *nothing but a complete mastectomy with surgery, radiation, and chemotherapy,* I was overwhelmed. My gut said my health would be compromised forever, if I even survived the treatment. Again, this is my personal testimony, and it may not work for you. All I'm suggesting is please listen carefully to your body and soul as treatment plans are being made. When I do listen to my inner promptings, it always works out. When I don't listen to my inner promptings, I find myself unhappy later on.

Discernment Two: Raise Your Hope Vibration

Even if you're not an old hippie, you've probably heard the expression "good vibes." When it comes to healthcare, it's important that both your physician and your response to the recommended treatment raise your vibration, inspiring hope. A cancer diagnosis initially deflates your hope vibration, but your doctor can help restore it. The hospital, oncologist, surgeon, or clinic can usher in hope and a sense of support and camaraderie. Similarly, if a doctor, hospital, or clinic makes you unduly anxious or causes you to feel pressured, you probably want to take a second look to determine if you're in the right place.

Every day we interact with different vibrations from things we watch on TV, hear on the radio, read in the news, or experience personally. Discerning vibrations is an important life skill. In a movie, don't you often feel your heart race just before a white-knuckle scene? Often the music builds up to intensify the dramatic event. Similarly, we can get these gut reactions, during and/or after we've met with someone. We get signals when something is scary, off balance, or not doing us any good. These exchanges produce bad vibrations.

In the United States today the practice of medicine is complicated by doctors' well-founded fear of litigation. This is creating a scary vibration throughout our entire healthcare system. Because of the high cost of malpractice insurance, medical practitioners have to pay dearly. Many physicians live in constant fear of making a mistake and getting sued, and this is reflected in their decision making. Some doctors refuse to treat high-risk patients while others practice defensive medicine, ordering unnecessary tests and procedures to protect themselves against possible litigation. This is clearly a terrible situation for both doctors and patients. Fear and healing are opposing forces.

After my treatment in Mexico, I had to locate a California-based doctor for basic tests and referrals for insurance purposes. Since my general practitioner retired the week I discovered the lump (he closed his practice because of the high cost of malpractice insurance and moved to Nevada), I had to find another doctor—and quickly. Since my case was urgent, I was assigned to the first available physician in the healthcare system, a thirty-three-year-old kidney specialist. I went back to him after I had completed Dr. Rubio's treatment to see if we could work together.

He looked at my chart, saw that I'd been diagnosed with breast cancer nine months earlier, and remarked, "I remember you; so, you had surgery?" I said, "Not exactly," and he looked at me strangely. I explained that I'd undergone low-dose chemotherapy, radiation, and immunotherapy and that my tumor was gone. When I told him I was cancer free, he remarked, "You know it can come back?" He clearly didn't approve of my choice, and his response inspired neither hope nor good vibes. Suffice it to say, this was not a man with a winning bedside manner. Yet from his medical training, I probably sounded like I was making an unwise decision, and he felt he needed to convey this to me.

At that moment I was so glad I'd gone to Dr. Rubio, where fear tactics and tales of worst-case scenarios were not practiced by any of the medical staff. I could hardly wait to leave the kidney specialist's office that day. However, it was later pointed out to me that if this physician had officially approved of my treatment in Mexico, he might have made himself vulnerable to a lawsuit: more lawsuit fear and low vibrations. Our medical care system is in critical condition.

Recent stories in the news amplify this dilemma. A sixteen-year-old boy named Abraham Cherrix was diagnosed with Hodgkin's lymphoma. When he refused a second round of chemotherapy because of the weakness and nausea caused by his initial treatment, his family elected to pursue alternative therapy at a clinic in Mexico. This story became news when a Social Services worker stepped in and asked the courts to mandate the treatment recommended by U.S. doctors. A Virginia juvenile court judge ruled that they *had* to accept the treatment that the doctors deemed necessary, even though both he and his parents were adamantly against it. Can you imagine the vibration surrounding this situation? Fortunately, a circuit court judge suspended the ruling and ordered a trial—which should bring needed attention to this important issue.

The press is keeping tabs with him, and the alternative treatments are helping him at this writing. A front page article in the *Chicago Tribune* discussing how Americans are seeking alternative treatments, cited a study conducted in August 2006 by the American Cancer Society, which said "27% of Americans believe that the Medical Industry is withholding a cure for cancer to continue to increase its profits."

We need to raise our vibrations if we are to heal. We need to rise above the cancer and help others do the same. This way of living exudes a certain savvy. I'll never forget my parting comment when I left the dismal kidney doctor that day. "Have you heard of customized cancer vaccines?" I inquired casually. He replied with an arrogant, "No!" Undaunted, I fired back, "If your wife were diagnosed with breast cancer at an early age, would you want her to know about all treatment options before she underwent a complete mastectomy?" He shot back, "No, I wouldn't even give it a second thought. I'd recommend surgery, chemotherapy, and radiation." I declared, "Perhaps I'm a messenger. I had the cancer vaccine, and it has worked for me. I believe it's the medicine of the future...good day, doctor." As I left his office that day, never to return, I knew my blood pressure went up. I do wonder if he remembers me; I know I'll never forget him!

Discernment Three: The Power of Asking

As I've mentioned earlier, during your quest for what is best for you, it's important to interview other doctors, nurses, cancer survivors, cancer experts, caregivers, and anyone else who serendipitously crosses your path. Some of these people will have answers from lessons learned and can share important insights. Encourage their stories, especially ones that begin with, "I have a friend with your diagnosis, and she's alive and well today."

It's also okay to ask your doctor if you can delay a dreaded part of the treatment. I'll never forget my husband's words when the surgeon said, "This is a large tumor; we have to take the entire breast." Bryan questioned, "Can't you shrink the tumor with radiation and chemotherapy first?" Had the doctor agreed to delay the surgery, I probably would have gone along. I guess at the time, I was so put off by the scare tactics I just ran.

Soon after I was diagnosed, I flew to Cleveland for a weekend conference and sat next to a nurse on the flight. When I overheard her discussing a medical conference, I knew I had to engage her in a conversation. My opener was, "You're a nurse, how interesting. Could I ask your area of expertise?" It wasn't in the field of cancer, but I went on. "Do you have any experience with cancer?" She told me she'd worked with cancer patients in an earlier position, so I asked, "If someone has just been diagnosed with cancer and is awaiting treatment, should she be staying home and resting?" She matter-of-factly stated, "No, that isn't necessary. Once patients are diagnosed they need to keep their spirits up. Sitting around waiting for treatment can drive someone nuts. It's better to stay active." I breathed a sigh of relief, knowing that my decision to attend the conference, fatigued or not, was a good idea.

Word got out at the conference about my diagnosis. People approached me, and I freely asked questions whenever I encountered a nurse, cancer survivor, or caregiver. I wanted to know about their experiences. If they had been a patient, how were they doing now? Did they have any regrets? What limitations, if any, did they have since treatment? (At that time I never thought to ask what strengths had been gained.) Listening to them after just a few comments, I could get a sense of the worst or best part of each person's experience. I asked a lot of questions to help me prepare mentally, emotionally, and spiritually for the cancer arena I was entering. I wanted to be aware of what I was about to go through. Knowledge is power, so I spent this conference getting equipped with both.

Jenny was another woman in my networking group who had been diagnosed with breast cancer. She was also asking questions, in her fashion. She'd been watching PBS specials and doing a lot of Internet research. A former nurse, she was science-oriented and wanted me to explain my immunotherapy protocol. I told her, "I was given a vaccine to educate the immune system so my own body could destroy my tumor."

She replied, "That makes total sense!" She did, however, have a mastectomy and sometime afterward we were engaged in a spirited conversation, discussing depression and the merry-go-round of emotions that cancer recovery brings. Out of the blue, she said to me, "I'll bet you'll be alive in five years and I won't." These matters are in the hands of a Higher Power, but I admire her spirit and willingness to explore ideas that are different from her own.

Discernment Four: The Power of Belief

When fighting to save our lives, we all need to keep our minds focused on the task at hand. Here are two books that are sure to help. *The Magic of Believing* by Claude Bristol is a classic. The original copyright was 1948. It discusses how we have to cast our beliefs out into life, to create what we desire. *The Secret* by Rhonda Byrne is an updated version with a similar message.

Each day we need to wake up and believe in our choices. We have to believe in who we are, whom we married, our choice of careers, our inner circle of friends, and the principles that govern our life. When it comes to life-or-death decisions, we need to claim our power to say *no* to situations and people that would disrupt this life that we create daily, through the power of belief.

Remember my collecting evidence theory? Many of my favorite conversations are with other survivors who candidly share their unique points-of-view. Mary is a colleague who had a mastectomy plus skin-sparing reconstructive surgery. On diagnosis, her cancer was stage one, and no other chemotherapy or radiation was involved in her protocol. She didn't decide quickly on the mastectomy; she did her homework, researching on the Internet, getting second and third opinions. What fascinates me is what she was told by her surgeon prior to her surgery. He said there was a 99% rate of success. This absolutely blew my mind! I hadn't read about any cancer treatment with a cure rate even close to that.

Sometime later, Mary told me that in addition to being told by her physician of the high success rate with surgery, she had also read that statistic somewhere. This furthered my theory that we collect evidence to support our point of view and further us along in our beliefs—whatever they may be. This conversation also convinced me that there is some unknown (or known) force that guides our experiences and interactions.

Along these lines of belief, when I told Mary I was going to Mexico, she initially thought I was going to a holistic spa and afterward I'd return home for my "real cancer treatment." It wasn't until a year later that she realized I'd approached my cancer treatment from an entirely different belief system and protocol.

Here is where it gets tricky, especially with strong personalities—and they do exist among friends and in the same family. You have to support and demonstrate love for one another, even when someone's belief is completely different from yours. We are really all on the same team; we want cancer-free lives!

Discernment Five: Systems of Support

There is one thing for sure—no one gets through cancer alone. We need help with our diagnosis, protocols, and medical procedures. Our family and friends come to play a role they've probably never dreamed of. It's difficult to place all our demands on any one person, be it a spouse, parent, child, or friend. Why do you think there are so many support groups? No one is the same once they have faced a possible death sentence. I love the artistic perspective of Carly Simon: *You now have a broader range of highs and lows.* The highs have a quality that is more euphoric; the lows become darker. Depression can be deadly in this battle, and it's a reality every survivor faces at some point in the healing process—and often more than once.

Although your physician should be caring and empathetic, it's not his or her job to hold your hand or be your entire support system. Your physician is your medical delivery system. Don't be surprised if you fall a little bit in love with your oncologist, surgeon, or M.D. As patients, we often come to regard our doctors as something approaching a saint. It's natural to hold them in high esteem, but remember what they do, and don't expect more. If you end up with a saint, rejoice, but don't expect doctors to be deities. They're human, too, and have their own burdens to deal with. Your sustenance will come from your courageous spirit and from the love and support of your friends, family, and the sometimes surprising kindness of strangers.

When you are in the early stages of determining your treatment plan, it's important to have people who support your choices. The last thing cancer patients have time for is "selling" their loved ones on their selected treatment. Here is where I am so blessed to have my husband, Bryan. I'll never forget the moment the surgeon relayed the news about a complete mastectomy. The nurse was sitting by my side to hold my hand or give me a tissue for my tears while my husband was turning green as if he were going to faint on the other side of the room. Suddenly the nurse ran to his side.

Bryan's mother had been diagnosed with breast cancer in her forties, so he was getting a double whammy. First, he faced the fear of losing his wife, and simultaneously he was hit with the memory of his mother's illness. My mother-in-law, whom I never met, underwent a mastectomy in her late forties, and the cancer later spread to her brain. She died at fifty-two.

As I was making my decision to avoid surgery, Bryan was initially skeptical. But since a mastectomy had failed to save his mother's life, he let me choose my treatment plan and supported me one hundred percent in my decision. As I look back now, I really appreciate the fact that he didn't make it more difficult. I had well-meaning friends who were worried about me receiving treatment in a third-world country and seemed combative about the issue. Later on, with certain people, I learned to keep my treatment protocol and situation to myself and only confided in those who were part of my support system. I didn't have energy for debates; I needed to save my strength for healing.

Discernment Six: Watching for the Signs of Life

Did you happen to see the movie *L.A. Story*? The main character, played by Steve Martin, is looking for love in L.A. At one point he gets a message from a highway billboard sign, directing him to go back to his girl. I know that was just a whimsical creative device, but the universe does have a way of issuing these cosmic messages.

After I made my decision to go with Dr. Rubio, my next task was to inform my mother and close family members. As I prepared to tell them I was going to Mexico for cancer treatment, I knew I might be in for more well-intended warnings. I anticipated this wouldn't be an easy sell.

My mother is a realtor back in Michigan. Here is the scenario that was going on at her office while I was doing my research: She told Linda, her sales manager, about my diagnosis, and her first response was, "You know, Nancy, there are clinics down in Mexico having tremendous success. I know a girl with breast cancer who just got back—let's call her and find out more about her doctor."

When I got up my courage to make this announcement to my mom, she already had a brochure in her hand from a clinic in Mexico. I'll never forget that moment when I called. We were both astonished and had the same jaw dropping reaction... *Could it be the same Dr. Rubio?* Although the brochure wasn't from his clinic, I felt this was a significant sign, and I was certain I was heading in the right direction. When I first met Dr. Rubio, he asked if I'd had any prior treatment, and I said no. Then he told me, after an evaluation, that my prognosis was very good. Even with the large mass in my breast, he put the odds of success at between sixty to eight percent with his protocol. This was surely another good sign.

Prayer has been credited with working miracles, and asking for miracles is okay at a time like this. The signs of life will appear. If they haven't yet, please keep your faith strong, and, if you'll pardon an old cliché, remember that it's always darkest before the dawn. Say one more prayer; research one more article; *seek and ye shall find.*

Discernment Seven: Focus Your Mind to Stay the Course

Whatever treatment you ultimately choose, it's important to place all your belief and might behind it. You don't want to waffle or second guess once you've claimed your power and made your choice. When you find the right protocol and doctor, focus on setting into motion the positive outcomes you wish to receive.

There has never been a more important time to "fake it till you make it." If you have a disease, start imagining that you are healing. Don't place your energy in the illness. Put your energy into the cure. God, as they say, is in the details, and in this case the details are the treatment protocols. Place your energy in the miraculous wonders of the human body that naturally strives to heal and balance itself.

Getting Referrals

Asking questions can be beneficial as you claim your power in your medical situation. Even if you've already opted for a surgical solution, there are still important things to find out. You need to know, for instance, that, in the case of a recurrence, there are other, non-surgical options you can pursue. When given the name of a contact, be forthright.

Below are some questions that might be helpful:
- Did you have surgery, and if so, what type?
- Did you have another method of treatment, and if so, what type?
- What post-surgery pain and/or complications did you experience?
- How long was your recovery, and what were the rough spots?
- What were the benefits or positives?
- How long did the chemotherapy and/or radiation last?
- How long were you off work?
- If you had an emergency or problem during treatment, was your doctor's office responsive?
- How long was it before you were deemed to be "cancer free"?

- Was your doctor consistent in his or her approach to your case?
- Was he or she informed, interested, caring?
- Did you feel as if your medical team was "partnering" with you, or did you sometimes feel patronized?

This book doesn't diagnose or dictate what treatment to pursue. It simply asks you to claim your power and explore your options right at the beginning of any difficult health diagnosis. Be an active participant in the decision-making process that will affect the rest of your life. There are a few doctors who are in such a war with cancer that they throw everything in the arsenal at the disease, e.g., high dosages, radical surgeries, weeks and weeks of treatment, etc. Meanwhile, the patient has to live through the soul-robbing treatment and side effects. You are the captain of your ship: be involved.

CHAPTER 2

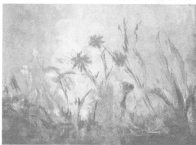

The Big Cut or the Cutting Edge

No one anticipates cancer, especially those of us who think positively and consistently practice a healthy lifestyle. I guess we figure that if we're living right and have our lives on track, cancer just doesn't happen. Okay, so I was mistaken!

My work as an author, speaker, and facilitator has always been both rewarding and challenging. I adore the satisfaction that comes from helping others and am always invigorated by sharing ideas with new people. This choice of profession has always made for a bit of an adventurous life. An active speaking schedule, coupled with travel and creative projects requires high-level energy, something I'd always been blessed with.

Not long after the 9/11 terrorist attacks, I was touring for my first book and began to notice a drop in my enthusiasm when I showed up for book signings. What was wrong with me? It was my dream to become an author—and here I am lethargically living my dream? I noticed I was tiring more easily and wondered if my thyroid might be sluggish or worse—that maybe I was slowing down now that I'd reached the not-so-sunny-side of forty. In any event, I expected that my lethargy would eventually pass, and I kept on with my demanding routine...until I got my wake-up call.

A Wake-Up Call on Speed Dial

It was 3:00 A.M., and I awoke from a dream. Strangely, I was positioned on my back with my left elbow bent above my head and my right hand on the base of my left breast. I'd never slept or awakened in this position before; I generally sleep on my side. Yet as I awakened, I noticed that my right hand felt as though it were lying on a rock. "This must be a dream," I thought, as I let this discovery sink in, and began to realize that, in fact, I was not dreaming. I had just found a large lump in my left breast.

I didn't want to awaken my husband, as he was working a second shift and had just started his night's sleep. Instead, I cried and waited impatiently for an hour, so I could call a friend on the East Coast and deliver my shocking news.

As disturbing as this discovery was, I instinctively knew I had found the lump "in God's time." After all, I'd had my annual mammogram every year for at least ten years and never had any abnormalities or alerts. My first matter of business that morning was a trip to my primary physician's office. He expressed platitudes of concern, "This is quite a large mass; whatever it is, you don't want to mess around. If it is cancer, my suggestion is to have it removed immediately." Over a six-week period, I cycled through the procession of tests. The last one was a needle biopsy, and I was told I would have the results in three days.

When the surgeon's office called, clearly it was bad news. The receptionist was frantically fitting me into the surgeon's schedule. Here I was looking at my planner, and I had business out of town that week. I asked the receptionist for the results, and she didn't want to tell me, but I insisted. Suddenly, she put the surgeon's head nurse on the phone. I quickly ran outside into my backyard and kicked my shoes off, so my feet were planted firmly on the ground. She began by saying, "We normally don't give the news over the phone." I replied, "It's been six weeks since I found the lump and I'd like to know." She stoically stated, "The lump is carcinogenic, invasive ductal carcinoma." I knew she was saying cancer, but I said, "Could you tell me again, do I have cancer?" She patiently said, "Yes, you do, and I suggest you pick up a book from our office before you leave town. This will help you prepare for your appointment with the surgeon next week."

The book was put out by the Susan G. Komen Foundation as a reference for newly diagnosed breast cancer patients. I was fairly calm after I got my diagnosis, before receiving this book. However, after a plane ride with the book glued to my face, I was certain that I would surely die. This book put the scare in me!

The fateful day arrived for my visit to the surgeon. My husband Bryan and I were nervously awaiting the 9:00 A.M. appointment, as the surgeon was running an hour late. He was a balding, gray-haired man, stern and to the point, clearly an old hand at delivering bad news. "Your cancer is advanced. You should have been on my table two years ago." The surgeon scolded as he continued, "You have no option but a complete mastectomy; the tumor is too large for anything else. And this is a high-risk surgery. There are no guarantees."

The message landed, B-O-O-M; like a cannon ball it hit me and thudded right into the center of my chest. The head nurse was standing by my side ready to hold my hand. I calmly kept a steady eye-to-eye contact with the surgeon, as I adjusted to his news. Suddenly the nurse exclaimed, "My goodness, her husband looks like he could faint." She rushed over to be by my Bryan. I was stunned by the severity of the surgeon's approach and message. I told him that I needed some time to think. He sternly counseled, "You don't have that kind of time!"

Had I panicked that day, I might have acquiesced to the pressure and quickly booked a date for surgery. But my earlier years as a CranioSacral Therapist studying massage, anatomy, and healing served me well; I felt calm and clear-headed. Back in those days, one of the statements I frequently made to my clients who were considering surgery for Temporo-Mandibular Joint (TMJ) or back pain—which I'd chant like a mantra—was this: *Make surgery your last resort*. Never having been sold on the-road-most-traveled brand of medicine, I was composed enough to know that I needed to get a second opinion and do some research. I bid the surgeon goodbye.

My third opinion came from an oncologist who concurred with the surgeon, stating, "After the mastectomy, we'll begin full courses of radiation and chemotherapy, then (if you choose) reconstructive surgery." I believe I asked for odds at that point, and this highly credentialed oncologist simply said, "There are no guarantees."

I left this ordeal wondering, *how do people survive the medical system?* As I walked out to the parking lot, I remember thinking that the only treatment option I'd been given (by these reputable doctors) was to endure the same procedures both my grandmothers had undergone thirty years earlier. Where was twenty-first-century medicine? We could go to the moon, transplant hearts, and train tiny robots to perform surgery—so many mind-boggling advancements over the last three decades. So why then, in spite of all the money being raised, had breast cancer treatment not progressed beyond the Disco Era?

Finding the Cutting Edge

Most people think diagnosis is a bad thing—quite the contrary! You can't begin the treatment/healing process until you are properly diagnosed. After many phone calls and hours of sifting through articles on the Internet, I called my minister friend, Roberta, for a prayer. Instead of praying for me, she gave me a sermon.

She told me about Dr. Rubio, who had treated her for a cancer tumor behind her eye, at his hospital in Mexico. When I had called, I hadn't even known that she'd been a cancer patient. My first reaction was knee-jerk; I pictured exotic herbs and coffee enemas. She assured me that Dr. Rubio was a cancer researcher, who had worked with cancer vaccines for over twenty years and offered more advanced technology than our FDA-governed scientists and doctors. His success rate, she said, was between sixty and eighty percent. She then exclaimed; he specializes in breast cancer!

I was familiar with cancer statistics—in the U.S. half the people treated with the usual cut/poison/burn therapies ultimately die from the treatment of the disease. I know that some reports now claim, thanks to early detection, that up to two-thirds of patients survive. But in the cancer arena, the common definition of "survival" is five years. What that means is that instead of dying three or four years after diagnosis, some patients are living maybe six to ten years after early detection. These statistics merely reflect the moving of the goal posts. Patients who live beyond the five-year marker are counted as "survivors," but that's little comfort to a patient whose cancer has metastasized in year six. Bottom line: It didn't take me long to reach a decision. If this Dr. Rubio could do better, I was interested in learning more—even if it meant leaving the country.

Dr. Rubio's hospital is located in La Mesa, Mexico, not far from the San Ysidro, California, border crossing. The day of my first appointment, I drove to an office five miles north of the border and was then transported fifteen miles by minivan. This meant I didn't have to deal with the risks and hassles of driving in another country. I was gratified to see that the hospital looked clean and professional. From the time I walked through the front doors, I felt a comforting sense of warmth and serenity. This place radiated a peaceful healing environment.

On first meeting Dr. Rubio, I perceived that he was a dedicated man, serious and kind. As we spoke, I realized that he understood the power of the body to heal naturally. He told me he had treated many patients who had already undergone surgery, high doses of chemotherapy, and radiation, all blunt weapons that destroy cells, healthy and malignant alike. All too often these treatments are far too toxic for patients to recover from. What he offered instead was a personally tailored vaccine that would enable my body to fight the cancer from within. In other words, my own immune system would destroy my cancer with this special vaccine boost.

Many doctors believe that once you cut into a cancerous area, the cancer basically runs and hides. Dr. Rubio explained that cancer cells are "smart" cells, and when someone cuts into the body to remove them, the cancer cells run from the incision site and wait, sometimes in the glands, until the treatment is over. Then they come out of hiding and continue to grow and develop, often metastasizing in a new area.

After an examination and review of my records, Dr. Rubio told me that because my cancer was so advanced, it would be necessary to contain its growth. My treatment would begin with low doses of radiation and chemotherapy—but much less than is used in traditional proto-cols. He didn't promise I'd keep my hair or be spared the skin-burning blisters from radiation, but somehow I got the message that I might bypass these known side effects. While receiving chemotherapy and radiation, both toxic treatments, steps would be taken to detoxify and fortify my body. I'm delighted that in recent years the development of less toxic, more effective chemotherapy medicines are keeping the im-mune system intact while they destroy the cancer. I know strides are being made in this area, and I'm delighted. I do suggest that patients ask questions about the known side effects of treatments being recom-mended, before you start in; also, stay informed as new medications are given or stopped.

No matter what treatment protocol you choose, the mind, body, and intuition *must be in harmony*. In my case, I needed to believe in the cancer vaccine and in my own ability to heal my body without the ir-reparable damage caused by traditional surgical treatments. As I mentioned earlier, you need to believe in your doctor, too, for he or she will become your partner in the battle for your life. I think many people act hastily when it comes to this important decision. A diagnosis of cancer, especially if it's already advanced, creates unparalleled pressure. So it's essential to take the time to find the right physician.

Weighing the Pros and Cons of the Big Cut

Most surgeons are good people who truly believe that the proce-dures they perform are the only right and responsible treatments for cancer. Surgery is their business, their life; it's what they've been trained to do. However, physicians with a busy practice and a personal life have little time to explore the latest innovative treatments and even if knowl-edgeable, they aren't necessarily equipped to perform them.

I had the opportunity to speak at a day spa that holds monthly edu-cational events for breast cancer survivors, complete with complementary spa services and refreshments. The staff works hard on these media-covered occasions, and the women who attend truly seem to relish the experience. What was interesting to me was the fact that the host was a physician, who specializes in breast surgery and reconstruction and whose clinic was located directly across from the spa. He even passed out a book to a select few, containing poignant photos of bare-chested women, some with one breast, others with none, and some with reconstruction. All of them had visible scars.

He was pouring over these photos as if they were works of art by Picasso. I thought my own God-given breasts, unscarred, are much more appealing to me than the variations of man-altered chests he was showing off that day. I do understand that a gifted surgeon's mastery of the blade is an art, and I don't want to minimize the lives that surgeons have saved over the years. However, on seeing those photographs, I felt more strongly than ever that women should be offered more treatment options that avoid or postpone surgery, so they have a choice.

How Could This Happen?

Remember my collecting evidence theory in Chapter One? Another incident that caught my attention was on a *Dateline* television special about a Minnesota woman named Linda McDougal. She had discovered a lump in her breast and was told it was infiltrating ductal carcinoma. She was so frightened by the diagnosis that she elected to have both her breasts removed and then simultaneously reconstructed. In her mind she felt it was wise to take the most aggressive approach possible. After her surgery, she spoke to her surgeon and found him greatly ill-at-ease. "There is no cancer," he informed her. Linda responded happily, "That was the point of the surgery, right?" "What I mean is," the doctor continued, "there was *no* cancer to begin with." Linda left the hospital devastated.

How this happened was a pathologist at a reputable lab had evaluated her tests and apparently mixed up her sample with that of someone else. Her story gets worse. After Linda's bi-lateral mastectomy and reconstruction, her implants became infected. Her next ordeal was emergency surgery to have them removed, and she spent the next three months in bed. Now disfigured and despondent, Linda no longer undresses in front of her husband; she doesn't want to take her thirty-one inches of scar tissue to bed. I realize this is a worst-case scenario, but it can and did happen. Although Linda's experience was extreme, biopsies are not always one hundred percent accurate, and post-operative infections are not uncommon. More reasons to collect yourself and investigate all possible options.

Are You Ready for the Cutting Edge?

As a friend once told me, *there is never a crowd on the cutting edge.* What is the advantage of this cutting-edge treatment, immunotherapy and the cancer vaccine? For me the vaccine meant that I could avoid the scarring and trauma of a mastectomy, as well as the sparing of my lymph nodes, a critical issue that is often overlooked. The removal of these nodes frequently results in *lymphedema,* a condition that causes the affected arm to swell painfully—for a lifetime. Although binding and exercising the arm may be of some help, there is no cure for this disfiguring and distressing malady. The side effect of lymphedema is not rare; it occurs frequently in post-mastectomy and lumpectomy patients. Elizabeth Edwards, former Vice President candidate John Edward's wife, was interviewed by *People* magazine. The article states that *after her lumpectomy, chemotherapy and radiation, she suffers from lymphedema, with numbing in the hands and feet. This was referred to as an often lifelong effect of lymph node removal.*

The final bonus with Dr. Rubio's treatment was that I didn't have to worry about lymphedema. Add that benefit to my list of *not* losing my hair, eyebrows, eyelashes, or taste buds. Early in my research I recalled meeting a surgical nurse who underwent the typical treatment of mastectomy, radiation, and chemotherapy. Two years later she still hadn't recovered her previous energy or quality of life. Of course, I know that building back the body after cancer and the radical side effects takes time. I just wanted to make choices so that I could look into my future and see my health completely restored.

An Outreach Call to Remember

After months of treatment, I was feeling desperate to connect with people who had survived this breast cancer battle. I contacted the American Cancer Society's Outreach Program. Once you sign up, other survivors in your area will call and offer friendly support. Within a couple of days I had two messages from cancer survivors. Rosie was a woman who, seven years earlier, had found an Oreo cookie-sized tumor in her right breast. She opted to have both breasts removed, to rule out any chance of recurrence. After her surgery, she underwent reconstructive surgery. I inquired, "How many surgeries did you have in all?" She responded, "Ten." And then she added, "I just had a consultation for an eleventh." Somewhat taken aback, I asked, "If you haven't been able to get things straightened out after ten surgeries, what makes you think this one will be different?"

With her history of ten surgeries in seven years, it appears that instead of really dealing with the mental and emotional components of claiming greater personal awareness and power, she opted to stay in the patient treatment phase for seven years. She stayed hooked on surgeries and doctor visits to distract her from the impact cancer had had on her life. In order to gain greater personal awareness, we have to *feel our feelings*.

I give credit to Rosie for her activities such as volunteering with the American Cancer Society. I think this service was her way of making cancer work for her by offering hope to other patients. Even though we only talked a short while, I gleaned a lot from her situation, and she reinforced for me the need to address emotional and mental health, as we revamp our lives during and after a cancer diagnosis.

Traditional Treatment Documented

Another speaking colleague authored a book from his detail-oriented perspectiveabout his wife's traditional treatment for breast cancer. He had endured his wife's suffering as the primary caregiver throughout her mastectomy, chemotherapy, and radiation. He found solace and healing as he meticulously recorded his observations during her nine-month-long ordeal.

His book was self-published within a year, and their story brought me to tears. It was the first time I comprehended how truly fortunate I was, hearing about their grueling experiences as she underwent surgery and high doses of chemotherapy and radiation. He detailed his wife's side effects and resilient spirit as she endured the loss of breast, hair, and taste buds. He also recounted their out-of-pocket costs that health insurance didn't pay.

With his written work of love, he went in pursuit of a corporate sponsor and struck gold as he managed to get sponsorship from a major pharmaceutical company that purchased thirty-five thousand copies of his book to distribute to families of cancer patients. These industry giants were impressed with the courage both he and his wife displayed, as well as the honest recollections detailing their experience. I was happy to hear of his success with the book and his new-found work in speaking to the related medical facilities where his book would be distributed.

After watching him tell his story at this private event, *I perceived something that was not mentioned in the program that day*. In spite of his book's success, his wife's condition wasn't so bright. Within a four-year period from the onset of her initial diagnosis, surgery and chemotherapy, she had had two recurrences: skeletal cancer and brain cancer. At the time of his program, she had just completed treatment for the brain tumors. As far as I know, she is still living, but she has endured three years of anti-cancer treatment, mostly chemotherapy to keep her alive, and has acquired an extensive hat collection to try to cover the treatment's side effects.

The impact of this illness is overwhelming, devastating, enlightening, and promising. Each healing holds a promise for a new life that is richer and more rewarding. I detail my own experience of turning this challenge around in a way that made cancer *work for me*—and hopefully for you. My focus is not *poor me, I may have a recurrence* but rather *lucky me, I have the inner strength to really move effectively in life*. These are the *treatable and beatable* tactics this book addresses. For me personally, the emotional and mental adjustments take longer than the actual medical treatments.

My breast cancer story and healing process took longer than a year because I didn't have surgery to remove the tumor. With the cancer vaccine, my own immune system destroyed my cancer. Here I am four years plus from my initial diagnosis, and I'm delighted to report that there has been no recurrence, no metastasis, and I've been consistently building my body back to be strong and healthy inside and out. (Utilizing all the methods I discuss in this book.)

I don't want to make immunotherapy and healing stage three breast cancer appear to be a snap or a guarantee. As you read through my personal story, you will see it took plenty of patience, faith, hard work, and discipline. The discipline should be with a capital D because it entails the dietary and medical regime and additionally keeping the *treatable and beatable* mindset—so I stayed focused on how to improve my life.

With this privileged story to tell, I invite patients and families to read about how claiming your power early on and making a decision based on your beliefs and disciplines can assist in keeping you alive. Every day I wake up and am grateful that I have my husband, my family and friends, my passions, my doctor, as well as my "girls" a.k.a. breasts, which all help me have a greater vitality and disposition. My hope is that if you or a loved one are diagnosed with cancer, you will take a moment to do some research and know your options. Whatever treatment you select, *here's to a great healing for you.*

CHAPTER 3

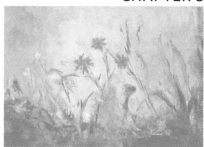

Know Your Options: The Cancer Vaccine

T he treatment option I chose to heal stage three breast cancer was immunotherapy, using a customized vaccine created from my own cancer cells. With the recent FDA approval legalizing the cervical cancer vaccine, we have just started to see cancer vaccines in the United States. Since this treatment is one you've likely heard about, but probably not in depth, I hope to shed some light. Let me explain in laymen's terms how the cancer vaccine helped my body successfully destroy the 3.5 cm tumor in my left breast.

The purpose of the vaccine is to create a cancer-repellent-metabolic-environment.

The vaccine works initially by removing the protective protein coating at the tumor site. It also educates the white blood cells to recognize and destroy the tumor and break it down without damaging healthy cells. This personally-tailored vaccine (which unlike a flu vaccine can be used in *your* body *only*) equips your immune system to overcome the malignant cells. It fights the cancer from within; it's an internal approach rather than an external invasive one.

In selecting this treatment, it's important to understand the concept that a vaccine has the capacity to be a potent immune system booster, teaching your body to destroy your own cancer. (More details on the several different types of vaccines Dr. Rubio uses are outlined in the Afterword section.) You may ask why do you need several types of vaccines if you only have one type of cancer. I'll use the analogy of exercise; just as we don't get optimum results from doing one exercise over and over, because the body becomes acclimated, we can't use the same vaccine repeatedly. If we do a variety of exercises, we get better results; the same is true with the vaccines. On an individual basis, Dr. Rubio discusses with patients which multi-vaccine method is most effective. This is because cancer cells are smart and will fight so hard for survival that they often starve off the healthy cells to keep themselves alive. The vaccine approach has to be even more aggressive to activate the immune system and stay on the offense. This ensures the immune system is always on high alert, ready to attack and destroy any malignant cells and keep the patient progressing.

You Went to Mexico???

So often when people hear I went south of the border for my cancer treatment, their imagination runs wild. When they think of leaving our sophisticated medical system in the United States to go to *Mexico*, they imagine back street alley clinics, unsanitary conditions, overcrowded facilities, and less modern equipment and procedures.

I can't speak for all the clinics and hospitals offering alternative approaches to cancer, but I can describe Dr. Rubio's hospital and how my treatment began.

The initial hospital stay lasted three weeks. Usually patients come for one to eight weeks (depending on the condition) to give the medical team time to contain the cancer while the vaccine is being cultured. What I mean by "contain the cancer" is that the traditional methods of radiation and chemotherapy are given in conjunction with health-building chelation IVs and vitamin shots. These protocols are followed along with detoxification rituals.

The Hospital San Martin is a small two-story professional medical facility. It is located in a residential area but has been completely rebuilt to accommodate the hundreds of patients who pass through the doors. Doctors and nurses, dressed in uniforms, are on staff 24/7. Each patient is moved into a private hospital room, equipped with two beds, one for the patient and one for family members.

Each of the nine private rooms has a luxurious private bathroom equipped with a bathtub, so that patients have a private self-contained space. Every hospital room is equipped with remote-controlled TV and CD players.

Plenty of educational videos and materials about cancer treatment are provided to help patients become educated during treatment. This is such an important aspect of the *treatable and beatable* approach; patients and families who want to engage their minds in how to heal cancer have a one hundred percent advantage over those who just let treatment happen. Read the books, watch the videos, and see what fits for you and what doesn't. Remember that you need to be an active participant during your treatment. Getting yourself educated, while your doctors are busy making the rounds, is how you take on this active role and reduce your stress.

My Treatment Kickoff

Dr. Rubio began my treatment with a three-day fast because I was physically strong enough. I drank nothing but vegetable and fruit juices the first three days under his care. Not all patients can start with a fast, but the purpose of beginning my treatment like this was to give my organs a chance to rest and detoxify before the chemotherapy and radiation treatments began. After three days of fasting, I graduated to all-organic meals that included fresh produce and hormone-free meats. Each morning began with a fresh vegetable juice. These juices would be a practice I would continue, long after treatment at the hospital. (I still drink at least three to five fresh juices weekly.) Another important detail to cover is that not only was the treatment less severe in Mexico, the food was healthier! The hospital diet was sugar free, an important fact to note because *sugar nourishes cancer cells.*

When I first began treatment, Dr. Rubio knew my concerns about chemotherapy and hair loss. I questioned myself; was I so vain that I couldn't stand to lose a breast or my golden locks? Then the hospital's psychologist validated my feelings when he told me about a thirty-four-year-old woman who had one breast removed, lost her hair from che-motherapy, and echoed those familiar words, *I no longer feel like a woman*. She lost her will to fight and soon died. Believe me, I know there's much more to being a woman than possessing a certain exterior, and I don't consider myself shallow. Regardless (like it or not), as part of the decision-making team, I knew my spirit would be profoundly affected by those grim side effects.

Dr. Rubio assured me I'd be receiving low doses of chemotherapy and radiation and probably would not lose my hair. The strength of treatments was about one-fifth the strength of what would have been administered to me in the United States. The reason I was given these lower doses was because chemotherapy and radiation are not the pri-mary treatment methods, but rather are used to contain the cancer (keeping it from spreading) while the customized vaccine is being pre-pared.

Because of my personal concerns over chemotherapy and losing my hair, I was never told when my first chemotherapy treatment was actu-ally administered. Initially this surprised me, but later I realized I was spared that anxiety. I had several IV lines going into the shunt in my chest, most of them providing nutrients to build and detoxify my body. I was also receiving chelation therapy, immunotherapy, and hormonal therapy, so I wasn't exactly sure when I first had chemotherapy. Later I became astute enough to tell what chemotherapy *felt like* and knew when I was having it.

Preparing the first vaccine took twenty-one days, and Dr. Rubio created it from my own blood and cancer cells. As mentioned earlier, he prepares a variety of vaccines because he knows how clever cancer cells are at adapting to their environment while they fight for survival. They may originate as a "mistake" in the cellular composition, but once they proliferate, they become extremely territorial. As I awaited the first vaccine injection, I continued with the chemotherapy and radiation to stop the cancer's growth and contain the tumor. But even after fifteen radiation treatments, I experienced no burning of the breast, nipple or the surrounding areas. I also kept all my hair, eyelashes, and taste buds.

I didn't realize until later on, when I read books about traditional treatment methods, how mild my side effects had been compared to those of other cancer survivors.

You might understand I was pretty nervous as I got myself ready for the first vaccine injection. In my nervousness, I began to question myself and my decision. Thoughts ran wild through my mind: *Will this vaccine really make me well? I'm already sick with cancer; now I might get sick from the vaccine? Can my body really withstand all this treatment? Will I ever be able to see another doctor in the United States after having done all this non-FDA-approved treatment down here?* Even when my mind conjured up all these sudden fears, I never once wished that I had cut the cancer out. The mastectomy option, from the beginning, was clear to me as the path I did not want to pursue. So when these anxieties would fester, I'd focus on the facts that I had found another way to destroy the cancer and that Dr. Rubio had been treating patients with vaccines for nearly twenty years. I'd coax my mind back to the thrill that I'd found a less invasive option and was able to save my breasts. Before I knew it, I was ready to get on with this Indiana Jones-style adventure!

My good doctor told me that the side effects vary from person to person. Throughout my preliminary treatment—radiation and chemotherapy—I never vomited. I had my share of nausea, but the medication Zofran helped to calm my stomach, so I never became violently ill. I wish I could tell you that the vaccine experience was a day in the park—nothing worse than the inoculations one gets before going overseas. In fact, I had very little reaction to the first vaccine, but they have a cumulative effect.

The initial vaccine was the mildest because Dr. Rubio was testing to see how much my system could handle. Each time he could revise the white blood cell count, either up or down, depending on my feedback. It is so important to give your doctors accurate feedback on how you are doing, so they can adjust your treatment accordingly. I don't recommend you tell the doctor everything is great, and then complain to family, friends, or other patients because you feel like c-r-a-p. If you feel awful, tell the doctor to his face and see if you can solve the problem together.

Progressing Through Treatment Doesn't Always Feel Like Progress

For the first three months, I received the vaccine once a month. With the second round I had more of a flu-like reaction. When I told Dr. Rubio that I felt sicker than before, he didn't seem concerned. He explained, "I increased the cell count by 100,000 because you are doing so well. I want to boost your white blood cell count to give you more ammunition. This will help to fight the tumor more aggressively." As I listened to his explanation, I thought, *at least he said I'm doing well.*

After three vaccines in a row, I had more than flu-like symptoms; I experienced a significant (for me) depression and about six weeks of nausea. This was a difficult phase of the treatment. I learned that vaccine number three contained a new compound called a *dendritic* vaccine.

After that powerful injection, I went three months between treatments, and eventually the interval stretched to four and five months. Approaching four years into treatment, I continue to receive vaccines in order to keep my immune system charged up, so no other tumor sites develop. I will maintain this protocol until the five-year mark. Reaching the five-year mark, cancer free, is something all survivors relish.

My dear friend Roberta, who referred me to Dr. Rubio, had undergone treatment for a tumor behind her eye. She received immunotherapy and avoided having her eye removed, which was what doctors were ready to do at a prestigious hospital in Los Angeles. She shared with me a special affirmation she uses, and whenever I became especially anxious about getting the vaccine, I recall her words. The affirmation went like this: *My body is in harmony with this vaccine (insert any treatment) and loves to do its job identifying what is me and removing what is not me. The vaccine holds the power of my identity to heal itself.*

This is a favorite affirmation that can be used before, during, and after any treatment. Having positive affirming thoughts in your mind is proven to assist the body. This cannot be emphasized enough: Use your mind as an ally when these powerful metabolic processes are occurring. This concept will deliver a state of healing to you. Affirmations coax our psyches to a place of healing, so our bodies can follow.

Clearing My Emotional Landscape as Part of the Treatment Process

Anticipating a vaccine and experiencing the actual treatment are two different things. Before receiving a vaccine, I would naturally feel uneasy knowing it would initially make me feel sick. For me the process was emotional, too, and tears were part of the release I needed before a vaccine treatment. I can't speak for everyone, but I needed to clear my emotional landscape in preparation for the upcoming immune system boost. During the early stages of treatment, these emotional storms were commonplace prior to, during, and even after each procedure.

Here is where other patients came in to be helpful. If I was going through a down time, I'd reach out to another patient, and it would lift my spirits. It was like we were on a roller coaster ride, just different cars. We'd all be up and down—back and forth. If I was doing well, I'd extend my hand to a patient on the low side. With each new round of vaccines, I had no idea how (temporarily) sick I might become. The unknown is often scary, but listening to the success stories and reaching out to other patients helped me to build the trust and faith I needed to get through.

I knew that if I expressed my emotions prior to treatment, clearing my emotional landscape, I would have more physical strength to fight during the vaccine treatment. During the intensive early months, there is an enormous amount of energy consumed as the vaccine engages the immune system in a defense-and-attack mode. This is a time when the battle between your immune system and cancer takes all your strength, leaving little energy for managing the challenges of daily life. Things like rush-hour traffic, paying bills, working, and running a household, all became difficult. Sometimes just cooking and washing all the dishes at the end of the day would be my greatest accomplishment.

In spite of the side effects from a vaccine, I knew that each treatment was strengthening my immune system and that the outcome was promising. After each battle was over, even if the side effects took a week or a month to subside, I was rewarded with renewed strength. It was about six months into treatment, when I received my fourth vaccine, that I really began to notice major improvements in my health and energy. The tumor had shrunk fifty percent in the first month, but the remaining portion took nearly a year to disappear.

As I was approaching my fifth treatment, I began to experience a profound burst of energy and purpose. I was even taking on ambitious projects such as closet cleaning, garage sales, and house painting. Now the trick was to talk myself into enduring another injection that was sure to make me temporarily ill. At this point, I forced myself to remember how *critical it is to continue the course of treatment* and not bail out early just because I felt pretty good. *Stay the course* was my mindset for success.

About nine months after my treatment began, I received what is called the non-specific vaccine, a.k.a. the "heavy-hitter dose." It was comprised of the highest number of white blood cells to date, with a specific component that included other viruses to strengthen my immune system further. When I went in for vaccine number five, I was especially determined not to let the side effects get me down.

Be Gentle with Yourself

The effects of the cancer battle, no matter what treatment you choose, take a toll on the emotions as well as the body. Like most people, I'm most likely to get down when I feel ill. It's then that I need to call on close friends and confess, "I'm tired of fighting cancer. I'm tired of feeling rotten. I'm tired of being tired!" I need to officially announce, "I'm the president of the Poor-Little-Me (PLM) Club. No one wants to join, but I'm still the President." I need to openly feel sorry for myself and just vent, rather than internalizing feelings of anger and self-pity.

For all my determination not to let the non-specific vaccine overwhelm me, I still had more lessons to learn. Perhaps the most difficult was to accept the fact that it wasn't smart to try to be Superwoman with Cancer. It was okay to feel down, depressed, and shaken up. Vaccines are powerful medicines, and I was not in control of my body when this cancer-fighting battle had been revved up. If I felt misery, fine; let's be real and feel, but maybe not dwell here. By acknowledging the emotion, I could release it and get it off my chest. (This is one of my favorite expressions now as a breast cancer "thriver.")

I was told by one wise woman, "You need to spend ninety-five percent of your energy on yourself and not take on the cares of others, let alone the world." I needed to view selfishness, which I'd always considered a character flaw, as something positive—a form of self-nurturing. I was also told to watch where I was investing my time and to monitor my energy. As someone who generally likes to help and be supportive of others, this was a difficult but necessary assignment. Cancer is a series of lessons on things you need to change or adapt to. I was in the school of healing, and my "teacher," cancer, was giving me plenty of life lessons.

With all of my body's vital-force energy being engaged by the immune system, my brain wasn't exactly functioning at peak levels. I did experience slight memory loss during the intensive first year, but this was very temporary. Again, I decided an affirmation was a good idea for bringing the memory up to rightful capacity. Here is my easy-to-remember affirmation: *I have a brilliant memory!* I love to tell this to people, and I frequently tell it to myself. When you're a fifty-something woman, people look at you in disbelief, "*You* have a brilliant memory?" I, of course, repeat it, to really get them going. Another reason that my memory statement is true is because I had a less invasive cancer treatment. No matter what treatment protocol you've been through, you want a *treatable and beatable mindset*. Here is an affirmation to support us all: *I have the right doctors and medical team to provide me with the treatment I need. My medicine is the best in the world, for my perfect health to manifest now.* Focus on these thoughts, no matter what fears are coming into your mind. If you believe you have the best medical team for you, you're likely to get it.

Protecting My Health by Protecting Myself

After receiving a dose of the vaccine, it's ideal to create a cocoon around yourself for a week or so, especially when you are in the early stages of treatment. This approach always gave me the best response to the treatment. Suffice it to say, I'd just had my immune system loaded up with additional soldiers whose mission was to destroy a tumor (or bacteria to compete with the tumor). I definitely didn't need a lot of outside stimulation, since I had a full-fledged war going on inside me!

For me this was not a time to go out in a crowd; my senses were heightened and could easily be overwhelmed. In the days following an injection, my sense of smell was heightened. Everything was amplified: sounds, scents, feelings, etc. The smell of cigarette smoke could make me violently ill. Treatment means it is time to treat *yourself*. If you have a partner who smokes, ask him or her to read this section of the book and to refrain from smoking at home during your treatment. Make the request that they wait a few hours after a smoke before coming into your presence. Still to this day, when people light up a cigarette around me, I tell them I've had chemotherapy and am very sensitive to smoke. It's just my way to let them know it's nothing personal, as I will usually walk away.

I also continually need to be sure my body is well hydrated, before and after treatment. The vaccine, in its mission to destroy cancer, needs to be flushed out of the system. Not only is drinking plenty of fluids during treatment important, but another part of the process is taking daily salt baths to help cleanse the body and flush out the effects of radiation, chemotherapy, and the vaccine. Since the skin is the largest organ of elimination, these daily salt soaks are an essential part of the flushing process. The latest trend to help detoxify the body is specialized foot baths, which draw toxins out of the feet as you soak in electrically-charged water. It works because gravity pulls the toxins to the lower extremities, and they get eliminated into the water at the completion of the foot bath. The next organ of elimination, the colon, needs flushing as well. Daily enemas were part of the process. Once you get the hang of this, it's not so bad. Now I think you're really getting the picture of why avoiding crowds is a good idea during this phase of treatment. (More details about these methods are in Chapter Nine and Resources.)

Hormone Blocking Factor

Another part of Dr. Rubio's treatment was the hormone-blocking factor. For estrogen receptive tumors, the production of estrogen has to be shut down, to assist with the tumor's destruction. For peri-menopausal women, what does this mean? It means immediate menopause! I don't care for the phrase *hot flashes*, so I'll refer to this physiological phenomenon as *temperature changes*. These temperature changes happen in conjunction with all the other fun stuff I just described.

Reporting side effects to your doctor is a very important thing to do. This is not the time to test your pain and discomfort threshold. When treatment side effects seem unbearable he or she might be able to make an adjustment or two. I know Dr. Rubio did adjust my Tamoxifin dosage after about nine months, when I complained. I described my symptoms as joint pain, weight gain, depression, and lethargy. Even when sitting on the couch, my joints hurt. I felt as if my skeleton had aged twenty years, not to mention the rest of me. I know so many women who have suffered greatly with hormone blockers. The point here is to speak up! If your doctors can recommend something, I'm sure they will.

Circadian Rhythm and the Importance of Sleep

Another side effect of the entire treatment—chemotherapy, radiation, hormone therapy, and vaccines—is the need for sleep. For several months during my treatment, I preferred to sleep ten to twelve hours a day. During this phase I wanted to remain horizontal even when I was awake. Getting to bed before 10:00 P.M. became very important in the circadian rhythm cycles that affect hormone production, brain wave activity, and cell regeneration. For example, at night during sleep, the pineal gland secretes melatonin. Several studies indicate that melatonin can boost the performance of cancer therapies such as radiation and chemotherapy. Melatonin is also said to increase radiation-induced tumor cell death. It also helps ward off negative side effects of chemotherapy on healthy cells and tissues.

Cortisol is another important hormone, which helps to regulate the immune system and support natural killer cell activity. It is released by the adrenal glands in the early morning hours, peaking at dawn, after hours of sleep. This helpful hormone has significance in that it boosts the immune system. Two variables dramatically affect cortisol levels: good sleep and stress prevention or coping skills.

What the Future Holds

In addition to immunotherapy, there are a number of cutting-edge treatments that may soon replace the traditional surgery/chemotherapy/radiation protocol, or at the very least, offer significant options. New therapies include precisely targeted radiation that preserves healthy tissue, radio-wave therapy, and angiogenesis blockers that inhibit the blood supply to cancer cells, causing them to starve. There are new chemotherapies that don't cause hair loss and actually help boost the immune system. These are all significant changes we need to be grateful for. But we also need to demand more; patients need more options and detailed explanations about treatment processes with this cancer explosion going on in our affluent modern-day society. Consumers need to make their needs known now.

Even though stem-cell research has been restricted at the national level, Californians have voted in a $3 billion budget to be used exclusively for this purpose. Some stem-cell testing has already been done in the cancer field, and with this new funding, the outlook is promising. U.S. researchers are intent on finding less invasive cancer treatments, and I know that Dr. Rubio and other medical pioneers have helped pave the way.

Whatever choice one ultimately makes, the decision about your treatment is a life-and-death matter. It's important to gather as much information as possible, survey a multitude of experts, and weigh the facts at hand. I know of one woman who got twelve "second" opinions; at the very least, you need more than one. I don't advocate that everyone follow my path and take the approach that worked for me; however, I do advocate that you consider all your options. I want you to know that you have power and a responsibility to yourself, to *use* your power when making choices that will affect the rest of your life.

That said, I'm well aware that as it stands now, medical choices to some degree are dictated by insurance and personal financial resources. I know that some of you reading this may not have any health coverage at all, or you may be limited to what your HMO or other health provider is willing to pay. If money is standing between you and the treatment of your choice, medical trials are one more option that might be affordable. If you are exploring treatments not covered by insurance, explain your financial situation to the medical team and see what can be worked out.

Don't let money dictate your health at a time like this. Nothing is more important in healing cancer than you believing in your treatment. I'll give you this analogy: Would you rather have a healthy body or a big house or fancy car? The vehicle we really live in and drive around with is our own human body. This is the vehicle that really influences my existence, so I spend the most money on it.

Since there is a whole lot of mind-over-matter going on with any cancer healing, why not believe you can have the funds for whatever treatment you need. If this is a stressful area for you, here are some affirmations to help you meet your financial needs and not live in fear of your medical expenses. Say these affirmations daily, and write a few of your own that really make you feel like you can have anything.

I open myself to a more abundant flow. I allow myself to receive abundance as a show of the Benevolent Power that is helping me to heal now! I have a large, consistent, dependable, permanent financial income now. I am blessed beyond measure; I am a treasure.

CHAPTER 4

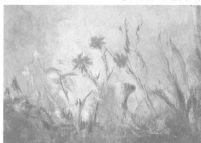

Taking
Time Out

Everyone likes time off, right? As patients and loved ones, if we allow ourselves some time for self reflection, we can go deeper into the healing experience. Here is an opportunity called cancer, which can provide you with greater self-awareness. The reason I can claim this so certainly is because adversity draws out of us facets we don't see in everyday life. It's like being in school, only the "cancer class" is customized, because each person has a different set of lessons to learn. In order to do your lessons, you'll want to allow yourself a time-out, a special hiatus when you sit on the sidelines and re-evaluate your life. It's not about how cancer changes your life; it's about how your life changes as a result of cancer. If you have the courage for quietude, you are sure to gain some precious knowledge.

While in the healing process, I suggest you try to suspend the beliefs and perceptions that you currently hold dear. Be open, willing, and ready to discover new beliefs about who you are and what you're here to accomplish. If, for example, you have been driving yourself pretty hard for acclaim and success, following all the tried and true formulas, maybe you have to redefine yourself a bit and use your intelligence to discover a way to succeed without driving yourself so hard. Or perhaps you are someone who has always given to others, supporting them in their dreams and allowing little time for your needs. In this process of discovery, if we don't attempt to control everything, maybe we might learn something new. In my experience, the re-evaluation process always provides the unexpected, if we allow it.

Taking a Turn on the Bench

As I considered various ways to approach the time-out needed for my healing process, I realized that I was being taken out of the game of life. The game of making money, enjoying a social life, networking, and aspiring to further my career—all these pursuits were on hold for a while. I marveled at the "timing" of my cancer diagnosis. After years of preparation to become a professional speaker and writer, I was starting to hit a nice stride of business acumen and customer satisfaction. Why was I being given a time-out now? Ask anyone who has started a business; they know what it takes to succeed and how hard it is to have to step aside just when things are finally starting to roll.

I knew I had to find a way of making the most of this less-than-welcome time-out, so I thought about professional athletes and what they go through while training for their sports. Here I was, trained in the "sport" of communication, and suddenly I was being sidelined. My new field position was the bench. I believe this "bench time" can be a critical phase in the recovery process. While we're sitting on the bench, we can observe others and how they play. We can also take stock of our competition. (Here is an opportunity, while we're waiting to perform again, where we can do what Olympic athletes advocate.) We can clearly visualize our success as we plan our next course of action.

Rest-Recovery-Discovery

Anyone with a serious illness knows you must rest in order to recover. For some, this can be the most painful part of their cancer therapy. I know initially it was for me, because I'm a typical high-achiever. If my self-esteem depends on what I accomplish, how would I see myself in an unproductive state, not to mention physically challenged? Not pretty thoughts, I'll tell you. Not only was I *hard on myself* early in my recovery, but I found my feelings reflected in a society where we're valued for hard work. Our culture promotes productivity, competition, and *results*. In the United States, we work longer, sleep less, and take fewer vacation days than citizens in most other countries.

A fellow "thriver," who saw that I wasn't slowing down much during my early months of treatment, asked one day, "Have you done any grief work around your diagnosis?" I knew what she meant. She was referring to the process of acknowledging feelings such as *why me?* along with the associated anger, sadness, and fear.

No sooner had she spoken the words than I found myself raging and crying simultaneously. It was horrible, but necessary. Her observation somehow removed the pin from the grenade I'd been carrying around inside of me. (Probably since the moment I was diagnosed.) Here I was with more than two decades of experience as a CranioSacral therapist. I had helped hundreds of people facilitate emotional and physical healings. Yet when it came to my own condition, I was just as stuck as anyone else.

I know very well how unexpressed emotions can create blocks, but still I needed someone to help me get real and quit dancing around the bench. This *Divine Intervention* from my friend was the beginning of settling in on the bench and accepting my well-deserved time-out.

I took a look at my business to see how long I could afford to take a leave of absence. I canceled appointments and put my assistants on hold. I said *no thank you* to networking events and discontinued marketing and sales efforts. Mind you, it was three months into my cancer treatment before I finally began to cut back. The question I tearfully asked myself was—*Carolyn, what disease do you have to get in order to allow yourself some time off? Isn't cancer serious enough?* Of course, the answer was *yes*. But it still took some coaxing to really pare down my schedule and take time out to retreat into what I like to call the *cancer cocoon*.

Purification and Progress

You really know the "cancer class" is in session when you are triggered into flashbacks. I still had some remnants of pain from my childhood that twenty years of working on hadn't quite healed. When I made the decision to embrace my cancer as a rite of passage, I needed to revisit issues I thought were already resolved. Toxic memories flooded my body and mind one more time. Anger weakens the functioning of the cells, so getting rid of anger is a huge and necessary step. When you're releasing stored-up toxic anger, it feels unhealthy during the process. Spiritual leaders, such as the Hawaiian *Kahunas*, see it as a form of purification.

Most people, when they begin to relive toxic emotions, stop the time-out and try to refocus themselves with more positive thinking. But this is *not* how the purification process happens. When painful issues arise, it's best to accept and deal with them. Don't try to embellish them, but rather let yourself review them one more time, like you're watching a movie. Allow these important issues to be released one more time. See if you can free yourself from past conditioning or ties that bind you in a stranglehold. In purification, we want to release and let go. If we give up the emotional ties to the painful parts of our past, we can prepare ourselves for the newness ahead.

Serendipity

Around the time I resigned myself to sitting on the bench, Terry, a longtime family friend, offered me her home in Palm Desert as a healing retreat. It was a win-win situation, as her house needed a visitor, and I was getting antsy with all the time at home. I wanted to start on this book, but felt uninspired. My husband Bryan had also been through a lot. Part of my home program involved him helping with IVs, giving me daily vitamin shots, doing all the grocery shopping, helping prepare my weekly selection of supplements/medicines, and morale support galore. I knew he needed a break from the caregiver routine too. I took my friend up on her offer, packed up the car with all my medicines, organic foods, research materials, and off I went.

There I was in the desert, with no TV, no contacts, and away from my office phone—finally! At first I was depressed, isolated, and bored, and I escaped by losing myself in sleep. Then one day I discovered a place nearby where they had therapeutic mineral waters. I began to go there each day, and these excursions provided me with a new sense of adventure.

One fateful afternoon, as I was stepping into the hot mineral pool, I was stunned by a woman who hollered—for all to hear—"What the hell happened to your arm?" She brought everyone's attention to the marks on my left arm—a memento of the cancer vaccines. I responded, more or less automatically, that my arm bore scars from a vaccine. Not one to go quietly, this lady-from-hell persisted, "Where on God's earth are you traveling to that you had to get so many—*'cause I don't ever want to go there!*" I wondered what etiquette advice Miss Manners would offer in this over-the-top situation, and *voila,* I came up with a perfect conversation stopper: "There are vaccines for reasons other than travel, my dear." End of story.

I felt a bit better but still self-conscious as I entered the pool and moved as far away from this obnoxious woman as possible. I nervously began chatting with the girl beside me, who said she was visiting from Alaska. When I inquired if she was vacationing, she replied that she was in town for a funeral. She explained her friend and former co-worker from the National Park Service in Alaska had met with a fatal hiking accident in the mountains above Palm Springs. Bryan and I always love traveling to the national parks and enjoy the people who hang out there, so I listened with great respect. She talked about what an incredible, healthy, well-loved guy her friend had been and how he'd suddenly fallen while hiking on a familiar trail and "hiked to heaven" all alone one day. I knew she was facing adversity, and I felt a bond as we talked. It was then I confided to her that I was recovering from breast cancer, which is why I had the marks on my arm.

Just as I got that off my chest, a very energetic, eighty-two-years young lady joined us in the mineral waters. Since there were no open jets available, she stayed on the steps and began talking to my new friend. This woman named Rehanna immediately engaged in the conversation and focused on my new friend, speaking to her with profound wisdom about the various stages of grief.

I was fascinated by this uniquely-named lady Rehanna. As I listened to her generous and loving words, I took them in as if she were speaking directly to me. As enjoyable as this interaction was, I selfishly began hoping that this wise lady would pay some special attention to me. A moment later, as if reading my mind, she looked over and said, "I'm off to the sauna." Taking this as an invitation, I offered to join her.

I felt a bit awkward as I followed this woman I barely knew into the sauna. But she immediately put me at ease. Her words were supportive, loving, and kind. She was obviously a teacher, minister, or healer and someone I was thrilled to meet. Our conversation continued long after our sauna, and we dined together that evening.

These are the mysteries and serendipitous moments that occur if we allow ourselves to be open and flexible during our time-out. If you meet a fascinating stranger, don't be afraid to engage in conversation with them. Live in the moment, and if something lifts your spirit, dive in and enjoy. My fortuitous meeting with Rehanna was a validation of how true this is and how important this phase of recovery can be. I love the expression, "When the student is ready, the teacher will appear!" The more hoops one goes through to get a time-out or find a special retreat, the greater the pay-off.

Don't Forget to Breathe

Rehanna's words to me that first night were, "You've got to clear out the old patterns, clear your channel, so you can heal and shine." One of the healing modalities she practiced was transformational breath work. That night, as we left the restaurant, she pointed to the place in my body where my breath was blocked. When she isolated the area below my rib cage, it felt empty and lifeless. I realized that often we don't recognize certain deficiencies until the right teacher, healer, or prophet comes along. In this case, it was a gift she gave me the first night we met.

I threw caution and skepticism to the wind as I scheduled my first transformational breath session, overcome at that moment by a wave of nausea. Granted, it isn't uncommon for a recovering cancer patient to have some queasiness, but until I picked up the phone to place the call, the nausea and anxiety were not present. I ventured a guess, based on my body of knowledge, that this would be an important part of my recovery process because my resistance was so intense.

Life Is About Working Through Our Resistances

As a researcher, I've often observed this *resistance phenomenon*. When we're about to embark on a new level of awareness and release old patterns and perspectives, these patterns, at whatever level they reside, create a great weight of resistance and fear. We don't want to let go of our beliefs, for we have ingrained responses from years of believing that something is true. When we're about to cut these systems loose, they stick like glue. This is what was creating my discomfort as I prepared to have a session with Rehanna.

Before the breath work began, she said, "All of life is about working through and accepting our resistance." As she demonstrated the type of breath that I would take non-stop for a while, I had some profound moments of fear and felt—*I have to stop!* All I was doing was continuous breathing mind you, but more nausea and fear arose as I struggled to work my way through it.

Rehanna facilitated the session with some hands-on work, using pressure points to help me release the pain. As I was laboring away with the breathing, I began to feel the soreness in my body subside. I'd been getting regular massages, and often these treatments would make me aware of areas of tension and pain, but they'd done nothing to alleviate them. This breathing process was touching on something deeper, and in this two-hour transformational session, parts of me were freed up in a most amazing way.

Afterward, Rehanna recommended that I take one hundred continuous breaths at the beginning of each day. These breaths are to be taken non-stop; you bring the breath in and release, breathe in and release. Soon after the rib cage constriction began to leave my body, I noticed that I was taking deeper breaths to the belly, and I began to experience a sense of aliveness. Happily, I still have the ability to breathe deeper and more freely today, just one more benefit of my time-out.

For me, this experience ushered in hope and the beginning of new energy and a sense of healing joy.

A Retreat to Remember

I often begin my speeches with the question: Are you interested in achieving your goals without diminishing your health and close relationships? I was facilitating a personal retreat in Hawaii for an accomplished entrepreneur named Lisa. She had heard about my retreats in Hawaii, and she herself was in the throes of chronic fatigue syndrome and numerous other afflictions. After meeting me a couple of times, she immediately signed up to go to Hawaii.

Once in the land of Aloha, she began reciting a substantial list of health woes and the alternative approaches she was using. The question I had as I listened to Lisa's laundry list of symptoms was: How could this woman write so many books and run a successful company when she had all these substantial maladies? Her chronic conditions were clearly a warning that she'd be wise to slow down and take some time out. However, her response to this health crisis, was to become compulsive about trying to *fix* it. Rather than doing something simple like slowing down or taking a sabbatical from work, she went on a high-flying search for a "quickie fixie" so she could continue her fast-paced career.

There Is No Going Back

One thing Lisa, this type-A lady, kept ruminating about was her "old life" before she developed chronic fatigue syndrome. She kept emphasizing, "I want to go back to where I was before I got sick." That is like Dorothy from *The Wizard of Oz* saying, I want to go back to Kansas and forget I ever saw the land of Oz. Each trial, even if it feels debilitating, has gems and jewels to offer. Once you've had a chronic condition, *there is no going back*. Living in the past and fantasizing about how good it was doesn't propel us forward. As we rebuild our bodies so that we are healed, we are ahead of where we were before diagnosis.

Please don't ever say, *I just want my old life back.* At some level your old life got you to the point where you became sick, so I urge you to try and not repeat that scenario.

After listening to Lisa one night, I went back to my room and realized that her definition of a successful life was clearly not my idea of success. I don't want to live my life as a high-performance robot by day, only to short circuit at night. Her determination to fix herself made me flash back to earlier years. I had actually lived that short-circuit-style life once, a long time ago. That is why she chose me to work on these issues with.

Pay Attention to Early Patterns

When I first moved to the West Coast, I worked as a catering director at a California State University campus. Early on in my catering position, I told myself that someday everyone on campus was going to know who I was; I was going to give them the best receptions, luncheons, and parties they'd ever seen.

There was an amphitheater on campus that held summer concerts, so I approached my employer and asked, "Who does the catering for the entertainers and concert promoters? Do you mind if I go after this business?" With his blessing and a few sales calls, I got my wish. Now my clients ranged from all parts of the campus community and included entertainers such as Robin Williams, George Benson, James Taylor, and Natalie Cole.

After three years of maintaining this high-profile catering business day and night in my mid-twenties, I became that robot who short-circuited after hours. Managing both my ambition and my health had become a challenge for me, too. It was no accident that Lisa wanted to work with me on her burnout issues. For me, Lisa was like a mirror showing me my own character flaws, how far I have come, and how far I have to grow.

Don't Pressure the Healing Process

Our society is so instant-gratification oriented, especially when it comes to getting out of pain and healing. We expect an A–Z overnight approach to conditions that clearly have taken years to develop. In actual healing terms, the reality is slow, one letter at a time—A, B, C, D, and sometimes you get stuck in one place for a while. The biggest shifts are usually foreshadowed by a *stuck* feeling, which is often a period of gestation. Then, once we're ready to move forward, we experience a rapid-fire progression of healing from the reservoir of strength we have built up to propel us forward.

Our lives, sooner or later, are going to reflect our values, for aging has a way of making us face the truth. Eventually our lifestyle choices and actions will show up in our physical condition and our mental outlook. A–Z healing takes a lifetime really, because by the time you complete all the lessons of growth, you don't stay on the letter Z the rest of you life. You are ready to shift to a whole new alphabet.

We've all worked with people who are highly ambitious and clearly run themselves into the ground. It's just hard to watch someone you love do that, especially if you live with them. But watching someone rebuild and re-evaluate his or her life after a serious challenge, such as cancer, is a beautiful and worthwhile thing to behold. It seems our society conditions us to strive for material success and beautiful things. However, the evolution of human potential, once unleashed, makes material success pale by comparison.

Scheduling Balance

So how do we find this greater self-awareness? How can we get our lives in balance and regain our health—without losing our status or success? My first suggestion is to have a special place where we can restore, relax, and renew. This has never been more important. Do you have one? Where is your special place? If you don't have an answer, find one! (This is a lovely assignment, by the way.)

For years, I've been a frequent visitor to Hawaii. This is truly a place that nurtures my soul, and when I'm there, I feel the greatest sense of inner peace. Every trip I make is filled with anticipation because I always leave the Hawaiian Islands a changed and better person. I think this is a key to balance. We each need to find our own *power places*, where we gain greater strength and bring this power into our lives and the world around us.

In Hawaiian culture there are powerful teachers and masters called *Kahunas* who have attained this balance of power and receptivity. These men and women are thought to be in touch with sacred knowledge and are able to stabilize others who are attempting to restore their spirit. When I first heard about the *Kahuna* initiations, where they are in a life/death situation and must consciously decide to fight for their lives, I couldn't help but think of those of us who must fight to survive cancer. No matter what treatment program you choose, you must be able to accept that cancer is a type of initiation, a trial-by-fire, and be ready to do battle.

Extrovert or Introvert

The continual need to master challenges and conquer the world reflects a masculine or extrovert energy. The need to love, nurture, and enjoy life reflects a feminine introvert energy. Most people get off-balance because they think that the rewards are greater in the masculine arena, so they spend more time there, with only occasional periods of pursuing nurturing and pleasure.

The information age with work, just one text message away, has spawned a relaxation-deprived society. The huge growth in the spa industry supports the concept that we've lost our nurturing-pleasure time. As one spa director I know said, "We now have to schedule our relaxation, or we won't get it." So we go to spas and seek nourishment for our weary spirits (and pay top dollar) because we're all so caught up in the race for glory and success. And when we become too dedicated to the fast track, we sometimes get a "time-out" from life called cancer. I know this is clearly what happened to me.

Earlier I mentioned Lisa, the work-driven lady with serious chronic fatigue, who kept exerting herself in a masculine-oriented way, creating an imbalance in mind and body. In the opposite situation, some people are nurturing and capitalize on pleasure in life, but they lack self-esteem, initiative, and the focus to accomplish their goals.

One woman I met experienced this scenario, but before she suffered any consequences, she was able to correct the imbalance. Maria was married to an entrepreneur who worked hard and played lavishly. As a family, they traveled the world, lived in a fine home, and had impressive friends. Maria appeared to be overshadowed by her dominant husband and obsessed with her twin sister's wealth. A sibling rivalry in full-force! When she spoke of the imbalance in her life, she voiced the fear that once her son reached adulthood, she might lose her only avenue of power and become totally submissive to her husband's whims and schedules. Just as the over-achiever needs to slow down and take a break, those who aren't challenging themselves enough need to shore up their inner strength and learn to demonstrate courage and assert their power.

In the case of Maria, she decided to start her own business, bringing healthy-food vending machines into the schools for kids. Here she was expressing her natural nurturing side with a commercial endeavor. She knew she was heading in the right direction when her concerns about her husband and sister just melted away. A funny thing about life balance: When we feel good about ourselves, we are less critical of others.

Redefining Happiness

Self-care is one of the keys to happiness. This involves knowing how to savor the good times. It's important to ingrain these moments in your memory and keep them alive; that way, when painful challenges arise, we have these happy memories to retreat to. We also need a creative capacity to make the most out of our difficult times. It's not the events in our lives, but how we react to them, that will determine the outcome.

I can't think of any better role model for this concept than the late Christopher and Dana Reeves. As everyone knows, a riding accident left the *Superman* actor confined to a wheelchair. In his early years of paralysis, he would tell his wife, Dana, "I'd gladly trade places with any bum on the street just to be able to walk again!" However, years later he told her, "I wouldn't trade my life with anyone." Clearly, he had a major time-out after his accident as he adjusted to his new circumstances. He came back at life paralyzed, with more determination to make a difference in the world than many of us will ever muster. Can you do the same? See your health challenge as a new way to appreciate life.

Spontaneous Regression

During my cancer healing I had several experiences of spontaneous regression. Let me explain what that means and then tell you why I mention it. Spontaneous regression (not to be confused with spontaneous *remission*) involves being triggered in the moment to an incident in the past. In recalling, you are still in the moment, remembering and regressing, and you go back to the past and relive it at a primal level. You not only experience memories, but you can feel the state of your being, your awareness.

The actor and activist Robert Redford said something profound when he was awarded an AFI Arts and Entertainment Award for his thirty-year career in film. I've admired his work for years, but his acceptance speech was singular and exceptional. He stated, "In all my years working as an actor, I always stayed focused on the road ahead; the next project, the next goal. However, receiving this award and going through old film clips and sequencing my career's progression, has caused me to look back, instead of focusing on my next project. I fully appreciate how worthwhile this process has been, just simply looking back, in the rear view mirror, so to speak."

Healing cancer can be a time of compiling the significant clips of our own lives and then reviewing them. Some moments are pleasant, others are not, but they are all necessary. This process of regression and going back does take work, and it's a solo journey too.

During my recovery process, I ran into a former coaching client who asked to schedule a session. We spoke briefly about her lack of a relationship, and she admitted that she knew she was preventing a relationship from becoming a reality. At her next appointment she confessed, "I didn't do the homework you gave me. It appears I don't want to look at the truth about myself—it's easier to just stay busy."

So many people have this mindset—it's too hard to find a relationship, to be successful, to get healthy, it's too difficult to sit still, or to look back and remember, so they go through life unfulfilled. They rationalize that some areas of their lives *are* working, so let's just ignore the ones that aren't. Yet deep down, this client knew she was keeping Mr. Right away, and she disclosed her loneliness to me. When someone says *sometimes I'm a little lonely*, it's usually an indication of something far deeper.

Loneliness on the Bench

Loneliness isn't fun and it isn't always easy to admit to. But if we finally confide in someone about what we are going through, it can help initiate the healing process. Being taken out of the game and given a time-out has a loneliness component to it, no doubt. We're no longer in the mainstream; our phone stops ringing, and our calendars aren't full, except for medical appointments. Because we are slowed down, there is time to remember, process, and reflect.

Stillness is a great gift, essential for contemplation. The ability to sit on the bench when others are playing at the very thing we love is a whole new discipline. As the famous Green Bay Packers coach Vince Lombardi once said, "It's easy to believe in yourself when you're winning, but to have faith in yourself when you're not winning; that's the sign of a great player."

With the exception of family members or close friends, people who haven't been through cancer can't really appreciate the physical discomfort or scary times we face alone in the cancer recovery process. But the loneliness does pass, and the scary times do subside; somehow, the will to fight for your life becomes a shining demonstration of your courage. You are making your statement in this world, just by staying alive.

You Deserve This Precious Reprieve

I know that some of you are going to have to stretch in order to create special time for yourself. You may have children, an aging parent, demanding bosses, partners who won't recognize that you need a reprieve—or all of the above. You have to ask these people, "What disease do I have to get in order to get some time off? Is cancer serious enough?"

You may have to enlist family members or a sitter to keep an eye on the kids or your mom. You might have to quit your job or resign positions in the community or church to create this space for yourself. The more hoops you go through to get this time off, the greater your rewards are likely to be. Taking yourself out of the game is actually the beginning of a new adventure—to greater self-awareness.

Cancer healing is a roller coaster ride, no question. Even with the *treatable and beatable* mindset, there are down times. I dealt with mine through the process of writing. My wish for you is that you'll discover some profound lessons as the result of this experience. I promise you the knowledge gained will change your life in a positive way. That's the ultimate result of the cancer classroom, which can be a significant transformer and teacher.

Tears of a Tumor

When you heard, did you think it was a rumor?

I found in my breast a large round tumor;

I wondered—why did the tumor pick me?

I knew I'd learn lessons before I was free.

Tears of a tumor, watch them flow

Not a time to hold back and stroll;

There is work to do when the tumor first arrives

That is, if you want to stay alive.

But inside this complicated disease

Is a new path of freedom and ease;

The lessons I will learn are my strengths and vulnerabilities,

The wisdom I will gain is to live how I please.

Oh, you shrinking mass, as you enlarge me,

I ask to always remember...how you set me free.

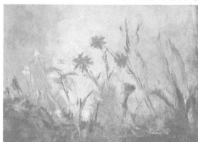

CHAPTER 5

Life-Enhancing Cancer

There are so many different responses to a cancer diagnosis: shock, disbelief, anger, pessimism, hopelessness, and upset to name a few. We all have some inherent baggage when it comes to the word *cancer*. At the worst, some feel it's a death sentence or the realization of their worst nightmare. Others see it as a bleep on the screen of life, like Merv Griffith, the former talk show host and entertainer. He has a totally positive approach to cancer, as an obstacle to overcome, just a temporary setback. Our response to cancer isn't a static thing; it bounces back and forth between two extremes, hopeful and desperate, and can include a lot of gray areas in between.

But ultimately we make the decision: Do we want a cancer that desperately dominates our life or what I call *life-enhancing cancer*? No matter what the nature of our situation is, we can use our mind as a powerful ally and choose our response. There will never be a more important time in one's life to evoke the power of positive thinking.

I'm not trying to minimize what we are up against. There is understandable fear associated with the "C" word and with becoming a member of its much-dreaded club. A recent article stated that one in five women would volunteer to have *both* breasts removed if they were diagnosed as a high-risk candidate for breast cancer. This may not shock you, but let me clarify this means twenty percent of women would *voluntarily* undergo *preventative* removal of both breasts because they *might* get cancer. They are so terrified of the disease that they believe mastectomy is a better option than prevention strategies, wait 'n' see, and careful screening.

Recent studies suggest that those who undergo any type of major surgery incur an increased risk of death—not just on the operating table—but for as long as a year or two after surgery. Researchers have already validated that surgery itself causes pain, stress, and anxiety, and when you add to that the burden of anesthesia and possible blood transfusions and hypothermia (low body temperature) during the procedure, it's understandable that the immune system is affected in a profound way. Some experts suggest that the combination of surgery and anesthesia triggers inflammation that can worsen existing heart and respiratory conditions, dementia, and, of course, cancer. At best, surgery is a win-lose situation.

Statistics constantly change, but in this country cancer is clearly getting to epidemic levels with a projected 1.4 million new cancer cases diagnosed each year and an estimated 564,830 deaths. Yet even with these numbers, most of our treatment protocols are more sophisticated versions of chemotherapy, radiation, and surgery, the same combination offered thirty years ago to my grandparents. Clearly, the "war on cancer" that was declared back in the seventies isn't even close to being won, but people are living full lives with cancer, longer.

Researchers have been exploring a number of alternative therapies, but often that research doesn't get into the practice of mainstream medicine. Instead, new and improved chemotherapies, new surgical offerings, and targeted radiation are the trend.

Happily, things *are* beginning to change. The good news is we are in a whirlwind of implementing several new breakthrough therapies, like vaccines, into our current medical system. However, for newly diagnosed patients, some 1.4 million people annually, there is no time to wait. Again, the Internet is helping patients to explore several treatment options and to select the one that will best enhance their lives during the recovery process, instead of being forced to endure the decades-old protocol of slash/poison/burn.

Healing and the Mind

Years ago, I remember watching the Bill Moyers' documentary on *Healing and the Mind*. One segment discussed cancer patients and the support systems available. The messages were profound. Many terminal cancer patients were taking on artistic pursuits such as writing and painting, exploring things they'd never had time for when they were healthy. When interviewed, these patients reflected that cancer had brought deeper meaning to their lives and that they were no longer so concerned with how long they were going to live. They were fully engaged in living in the moment and enjoying the self-discovery process. I remember thinking that this was an extremely spiritual endeavor.

Watching that program specifically encouraged me to continue my spiritual practices as I searched for meaning and success in life. I spent time in meditation, prayer, yoga, reading, and expanding my personal awareness. My thinking at the time was that all this would surely help me avoid cancer, and I could skip right to the life-enrichment part. So I was wrong! Now, as a proud cancer "thriver," I can look back and see that the most advanced personal growth I've ever experienced took place during my years of what I call *life-enhancing cancer.*

When I talk about an enriching personal experience here, let me clarify something. I think chaos is truly the great teacher. It's during these times of crisis that we cycle up and get new glimpses of ourselves, to discover who we are. I think of this as self-actualized living. A few favorite quotes: *Those who conquer themselves are greater than those who build up a city* and *If you want to heal the world, first you heal yourself.* Both are references to the potential impact from this life experience.

Reflection Not Blame

When I was first diagnosed, there was one lady who asked me, "Don't you feel that you have some unresolved stuff—that maybe you *created* your cancer?" Yes, I did have unresolved stuff, still do—who doesn't? But no one should feel responsible for *creating* his or her illness. Although stress may indeed be a factor, genetics play a role, as do environmental toxins—things over which we have little or no control.

This remark stuck some chord in me; there was a part of me that did feel responsible for my diagnosis yet was also perplexed. I was on track with my life, or so I thought. I'd graduated from the career you learn from to the career you live for. My former career in sales was respectable; I represented brand-name companies in the food industry, selling to resorts and their distributors. It was rewarding in many ways, but it wasn't my dream.

In time, I was fortunate enough to pursue my passion of teaching and helping people. The speaking/coaching business was something I'd always dreamed of doing. When I got into the speaking profession, I wanted to set the world on fire. I knew that for this to occur I had to master three areas: to be effective from the platform, offer a solid message, and make consistent sales. So I pushed myself and lived, breathed, and loved every moment. I set a couple goals early on: to publish a book and to become president of the National Speakers Association local chapter.

After three years of serving on the board of directors, I became president of the National Speakers Association in San Diego, and I also published my first book, *Staying Calm in the Midst of Chaos*™. When we were attacked by terrorists on 9/11 and life as we knew it changed forever, I knew I had a solid message that people needed to hear. I felt a sense of urgency to finish the book quickly and promote the heck out of it. This responsible, action-oriented nature is common in many breast cancer patients. We tend to think we can carry the weight of the world on our shoulders.

While I was promoting my book, I did a multi-state tour for Barnes & Noble, which included radio interviews across the country to help boost sales. All these efforts were in addition to building my speaking business and maintaining my coaching clientele. That's when I discovered the lump in my breast, which turned out to be a bump: a bump in the road and a reassignment. During my research on my first book, I met doctors who'd been rushed to the hospital with heart attack symptoms that turned out to be anxiety attacks. I realized that we're all vulnerable to overload and overwhelm.

Yet here I was a newly diagnosed cancer patient, with a life filled with so much chaos it was off the charts. Getting back to the idea that I may have "created" my cancer—our lifestyles and priorities are things we need to address seriously, but that does *not* mean we should add self-blame to our burdens. As I've mentioned, there are many variables, particularly genetics and environmental toxins, as well as some factors that science probably has yet to explore.

The point of *life-enhancing cancer* is to focus on what we *can* control. Our self-care and lifestyle, diet, exercise, and stress management are all before us on any given day. Please take this opportunity to make some necessary changes and welcome in a new approach to your life; this will assist in minimizing your chances of a recurrence. We need to safeguard ourselves, because let's face it, our twenty-first-century lives are complex and demanding. And yet no matter how much we safeguard ourselves, we can't feel like failures if we are diagnosed or a recurrence occurs. That is not the pressure we want to put on ourselves during this mysterious process of being a healthy survivor.

A great example of someone who used her cancer experience in ways to enhance her life is Dr. Wendy Harpham, a doctor of internal medicine who has received eight different courses of anticancer treatment since her diagnosis in 1990. Her story is so inspiring because during her initial chemotherapy, she asked herself, *How can my going through this experience benefit others?* As a physician, she had the medical knowledge to know what patients want and need, and yet with all her background, she couldn't prevent any one of her cancer recurrences. She exemplifies life-enhancing cancer because, while dealing with her own cancer, she wrote five books on various aspects of survivorship, all with the goal of "helping patients get good care and live as fully as possible." With her latest treatment, she talks and writes about the new and improved therapies, including the immunotherapy she has received. Based on her experiences as a mother of three, she also addresses the family issues involved when cancer hits a family. Through "knowledge, hope, and action" Dr. Harpham tries to make the best out of whatever situation she faces. I wonder how she would respond to the lady who asked, "Didn't you at some level create the cancer?"

Know Your Coping Style

During my treatment I had time to recognize the underlying coping styles that affect the mindset of patients and caregivers. I noticed through exchanges with family and friends that we all respond differently to crisis. I also became aware of the many ways people cope. I had already been teaching relationship strategies and interpersonal skills as a certified trainer for the *Color Code*™; this enlightened way of understanding our motives in life is based on the book by Taylor Hartman titled *Color Code.* Having taught the philosophy for several years, I decided to share his concepts from a slightly different angle to help people understand the different styles of coping.

As you read through these descriptions of four basic coping styles, realize that you may utilize parts of each one; but generally you will see one style that best reflects your approach to life. When reviewing these styles, see if you recognize yourself and your circle of family and friends. You may gain a better understanding of yourself and your loved ones by examining each description. Reflecting the concept that *all the world's a stage*, I've given them their theatrical posturing accordingly.

The first coping style is *The Superstar.* These action-oriented people rise to the occasion during times of crisis. They are natural problem-solvers and visionary thinkers who can foresee the necessary actions and then carry them out. In military terms, these are the generals and commanders. As patients, these people may be just as afraid as anyone else, but they keep their insecurities to themselves. They are intelligent and diligent researchers and will get several second opinions and even question their doctors if they don't see eye to eye. They are the true movers and shakers in the world and can be very independent during the healing process. They welcome support from others, but mostly they need to be surrounded by people who believe in their own power to heal and solve problems. These individuals can spend time alone and don't need much hand-holding, so they aren't the neediest patients—just the most demanding!

The second coping style is known as *The Producer*. People in this category want everyone to be happy, and they try to create win-win situations. In times of crisis they value relationships, so if they like and respect their doctors, they try to please them by being model patients. These folks weigh in the opinions of family and friends as they make decisions, and they find new friends wherever they go—at the clinic, the hospital, the pharmacy. As patients, they don't want to be alone, and they welcome and appreciate every kind of support, whether it be phone calls, visits, cards, or emails.

They work best by building a team, with a "we're all in this together" philosophy. As caregivers these individuals are great at rounding up the troops and getting things done; they're the friends who will make calls on your behalf, offer rides to doctor appointments, and keep your spirits up with thoughtful gestures.

The third coping style can best be described as *The Back Stage Manager*. Persons in this group need to view the situation from a peaceful place. They don't engage in a line-of-fire approach, and too many people in the decision-making process will make them uncomfortable. They are attentive listeners who will gather facts in a simple, understated fashion. They take their time making decisions and refuse to be rushed. They need to feel a sense of inner peace and certainty. And when they do, they are quite inventive and demonstrate great clarity and tolerance. Even when things aren't going well, they will be the quiet, uncomplaining patients or caregivers who stoically tolerate more tests and procedures with patience and grace.

From a doctor's perspective, these individuals make ideal patients because they are undemanding and "low maintenance." But these folks can also be stubborn. If you try to get them to do something that doesn't feel right, they're likely to dig their heels in and just say no. As peaceful and cordial as they are, they won't be pushed or manipulated. Sometimes they might need a little push to get them headed in the right direction, but as a caregiver you never want to use strong-arm tactics. A relaxed, gentle approach works best. Of all the types of coping styles, these individuals have the most difficulty making a decision. They may ask for your input, so don't hesitate to give it.

The fourth coping style is what I call *The Comic Relief Artist*. It's important for these people to keep things upbeat when crisis hits, or if life gets too serious, they'll head for the hills. They need some humor served up to offset calamity or complicated situations. These folks will be the patients making self-deprecating jokes, and they need the company of light-hearted friends. If you should find yourself a caregiver for such a person, surprise her with a picnic when she thinks she's going to the pharmacy.

Another form of good medicine for this type person might be movies and/or funny or suspenseful novels. If they're housebound, bring them some good DVDs and make a trip to a bookstore or the library for some upbeat entertainment. Laughter is highly recommended for life-enhancing cancer because it activates the immune system. When it comes to these fun-loving individuals, it's good to double the dose. They are naturally optimistic, so if bad news is in the air, be their personal cheerleader, because this is what they're used to doing for others.

Be Proactive

There are plenty of books on the subject of cancer; some of my favorites are listed at the end of the book. I read a few during difficult treatment months that seemed to give the message: "Your life as you know it is now over. If you win the battle with cancer, you must live the rest of your life following medical protocols, getting tested, and wondering if you'll have a recurrence." I didn't appreciate these books at the time, but if you can take the "your life will never be the same" message and spin that straw into gold, then you're on the track of life-enhancing cancer.

I believe we become more powerful as we face our challenges, as stated in the quotation, "What doesn't kill you makes you stronger." It works for me. Instead of embracing a message of doom, try saying to yourself: *My life is richer and fulfilled in this experience. I am learning the lessons of cancer and building a stronger mind and body. I am ready for perfect health and will allow my body to transform every cell during my treatments. I am a strong, healthy, resilient person.*

Be Active

For better or worse, I was raised in a very active family. Today this is our cultural norm, with most people juggling multiple roles, schedules, and overtime hours. But in the early sixties most Americans didn't live at this breakneck speed. My mother, however, was the Energizer Bunny, always on the go, so we kids had to keep up with her fast pace. Our days were filled with sports, piano, ballet, guitar lessons, golf, tennis, skiing, karate, Girl Scouts, and church activities. By the time I got to my teen-age years of high school, I never joined anything—I was too exhausted!

My strategy for getting a little rest and balance in my early life was to *play sick*. From time to time, I'd pretend I had the flu and get a couple days off from school and all my activities. Lying around eating bon-bons and watching old movies was heaven to me. It might surprise you then to learn that this childhood pattern was not to apply in my cancer recovery. There is a definite amount of down time and rest required, but life-enhancing cancer means taking on as many health-building activities as you can manage.

After resisting my mother's hectic pace in my younger days, during treatment I found myself inspired by it. I had to cook and eat right, exercise often, get together with friends, find easy and fun outings to lift my spirits, and meditate and pray to nurture my soul. I also needed to keep up with mundane chores like laundry, bill-paying, house cleaning, and moderate amounts of work to keep my business going. I remember wondering sometimes if I was pushing myself too hard. There were nights when I could barely stand at the kitchen sink. But I made it a point always to leave a clean kitchen to wake up to in the morning. It's a funny thing how the little things can give us a sense of accomplishment, when our lives are pared down.

I told Dr. Rubio how hard my revised schedule seemed, and he said this was good. In other words, we need rest and time out, but we also need to fight for normalcy in our lives: Making beds, cleaning, and doing the mundane chores makes you feel alive. Your life-enhancing mindset to improve your life, coupled with the courage to challenge and change yourself, will keep your plenty occupied while your body is going through treatment and renewal.

CHAPTER 6

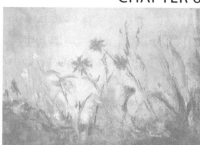

Learning to Fall

I n the last chapter I mentioned the importance of being active and maintaining normalcy. But as they say, *to all things there is a season, a time to sow and a time to reap*. Learning to fall is part of the letting-go process. We have to let go of the idea that we can *always* keep functioning at the same level while our bodies heal. When and how we surrender to the fall of perfect health is an important survival mechanism. We need to understand that cancer has some purpose in our lives.

Once we've explored our options and found our treatment program, claiming your power and purpose will help you move forward in a more significant way. Learning to "fall" and reprioritize are important issues when confronted by cancer. As Paul Simon's lyrics suggest, "You've got to learn how to fall before you can learn to fly." No matter how strong you are and how often you put on a brave face during a crisis, cancer will surely put some cracks in that foundation.

We All Compare Ourselves with Others

Just as I was getting off my motivational speaker high horse and allowing myself fully to experience the falling phase of my cancer ordeal, I received a letter from Kathy, a go-getter interior decorator. She stated that she'd recently been diagnosed with breast cancer and was now running a team for the Race for the Cure events. I was actively going through monthly vaccine treatments and decided to give her a call, to ask her a few questions, my first official interview for this book.

My instincts told me Kathy would have a "Superstar" coping style, someone who puts on a strong, brave face. Sure enough she told me, in a cavalier manner, "Oh, yeah, I was diagnosed with breast cancer, had a 3.5 cm tumor, stage three." (Her diagnosis was the same as mine.) She'd already had surgery, and I inquired if she'd gotten a second opinion. "What for?" she asked. "I trust my doctor; he's great."

After her complete mastectomy, four cycles of chemotherapy which resulted in the loss of her hair, eyebrows, and eyelashes, this decorator was soldiering on in her normal business mode. She admitted to slowing down and losing her taste buds; the latter was probably her major complaint. She'd also had a second, reconstructive surgery. So for her, everything was neatly wrapped up with a bow. Kathy stated proudly, "I took two weeks off from work and then was right back at it. It wasn't a big setback for me!"

Race for the Cure...Are You Sure?

With her hectic schedule, it didn't seem as if there had been any time to "fall" in her recovery. It appeared she didn't take time for the self-discovery phase I suggest in this book; instead, she *added* to her schedule by volunteering for the local Race for the Cure event, a noble cause and a great way for survivors and caring women to bond. I just have a question in my mind that doesn't go away. With all the Race of the Cure fundraising over the years and all these major companies donating their pink ribbon profits to the various breast cancer foundations, why has so little progress been made for non-surgical treatment options? Where does this money go??

During the interview, Kathy was proud to report that she was now busy running her business, volunteering, and happy to be an involved *survivor citizen*. She never mentioned anything about how the cancer experience changed her life or made it more meaningful. She didn't divulge any insights or details about how she was doing now. This exemplifies the Superstar coping style, someone who pushes through the experience with as few concessions as possible and divulges very little to others about their setbacks.

This approach is common in our twenty-first-century society. America doesn't know what to do with the infirmed or how to be the infirmed. We rely on our social network for support and approval, but when someone is seriously ill, many people disconnect. They don't know what to say or do, so they simply withdraw. If you need some assistance here, there is a section for Family and Caregivers listed in the back of this book. We're more dependent on our social environment than most of us realize, which is why, when we temporarily disconnect from this engaging world, it feels like falling.

You might be thinking, wait a minute, in earlier chapters you talked about the importance of life-enhancing positive thinking. Are you criticizing this Superstar decorator because she seems determined to help and heal? No, I'm offering an example of a woman who had the *treatable and beatable* spirit, but she wasn't initially changed by her experience. Kathy is a business wiz, and didn't see the benefits of taking time out or learning to fall, in the beginning. The point here is learning to fall can have its benefits, such as a renewed sense of purpose and awareness. I believe when we allow ourselves time to explore our vulnerabilities, in this situation, we become bigger and better people. This doesn't happen until we come to grips and become "real" with the situation. It's important to acknowledge our dark side, without lingering there too long.

About a year later, I kept running into this gifted decorator. I noticed she seemed to be always going on vacation. (Most hard-driving business people don't go away that often.) As years would follow, I saw she truly did go through a falling phase. She retired herself from the go-getter lifestyle and worked smarter. She had more time to pursuit travel and golf, and she allowed herself breathing space. No doubt about it, she re-prioritized and made some changes in her life after her cancer and looked happier for it. I call this a shift from cancer survivor to cancer "thriver."

When I was initially diagnosed, I responded much like Kathy; I didn't want to slow down and acknowledge any weakness, so I didn't. I was attempting to keep my competitive spirit alive, especially when one of my speaking colleagues, who had been through breast cancer, proudly boasted, "During my cancer recovery, I didn't miss a single speaking engagement." As professional speakers, these appearances pay our bills and expenses. So I, too, was determined to carry on, convincing myself that one or two presentations a month wouldn't hurt my recovery.

Medical Bills Are Not the Fun Part

In order for me to slow down, the universe had to step in and take away speaking engagements. Simultaneously, I was exposed to the reality that my reputable insurance company didn't want to pay for any of my chemotherapy. They only covered seven of my fifteen radiation sessions because I'd gone "outside" the system. This is not the case for everyone going this route. In my case, for my first year of cancer treatments, our health insurance paid around seven thousand dollars.

I knew I was falling when all this happened; the cancelled presentations and the substantial medical bills. Had I done the surgery/chemotherapy/radiation protocol, the health insurance company would have paid upwards of $100,000 or more. I knew at the onset going to Dr. Rubio would mean I would be financially responsible for all my immunotherapy vaccines and alternative health-building treatments. However, I was not expecting my insurance company to deny traditional treatment protocols when my PPO status had approved my claim initially.

Healthcare or Wealthcare

It is perplexing that some kind of resistance in the healthcare system doesn't readily explore these non-surgical cancer solutions. With over $25 billion poured into cancer research, the improvements are coming, but mostly with improved and modified chemotherapies and immune boosting white blood cell medication. They even offer more surgeries now for breast cancer patients; post-mastectomy you have several reconstruction options. It's true that there are new cutting-edge treatments on the horizon including the possibility of stem-cell therapy, and these prospects are very promising. But if you have cancer *today*, you're still pretty much stuck with the slash/burn/poison protocol that's been around for several decades.

A great deal of money goes into diagnostic equipment here in the United States, so we've become obsessed with early detection. But where is the money for less harmful and more effective treatments? Obviously, cancer translates into big money for the AMA, ACS, and pharmaceutical industry, as well as other related groups. There are some who believe our current cancer treatment systems are so profitable that the medical community hasn't been motivated to change it. It's always easier to maintain the status quo than to go through the turmoil of change. On the other hand, we are talking about people's lives.

During the falling phase of my recovery, I was angry that I had to travel outside my own advanced country in order to avail myself of gentler, effective, and cutting-edge treatments across the border.

An interesting study published by the American Cancer Society in August 2006 stated: "Twenty-seven percent of Americans believe the medical industry is withholding a cure for cancer to increase its profits." The study concluded that: "The lack of trust wasn't with the personal doctors, but with the pharmaceutical companies." Do you have an opinion here?

The realization of resistance in the healthcare system and the stress this puts on cancer patients affects us all. For me, the loss of expected insurance money for chemotherapy and radiation sent me into a depressed mindset. This was the part of the cancer process I didn't want to face. Who does? It was particularly hard for me, as a motivational speaker, because I'm heavily invested in the positive outlook approach. But now was the time when I had to succumb to the dark days, weeks, and months of fighting the cancer and my health insurance company simultaneously.

Dancing with the Darkness

I can best describe my experience as entering a vast dark crater that appears after a volcano erupts. I knew this hole existed in me when I was diagnosed, but in the beginning, I danced around it. I was busy convincing everyone that I was going to be fine and that immunotherapy was safe to receive down in Mexico. When I finally got tired of dodging this wound and realized that it was *not* going away, I reluctantly crawled into my dark hole and crumbled into a ball.

There was a lot to face in that bitter place, but it's there that I began the self-discovery process. Not knowing at the time if I would live or die, I reviewed my family life and relationships and assessed which ones were strong and nurturing and which ones I wished had been more fulfilling. I'd review my life whenever something triggered a memory and ask myself what was important about this person and/or event. So this next bit of advice is essential: Keep a cancer journal; it's vitally productive work, even though all you write may reflect depression or despair. In order for me to get this inside job done, I had to do some fancy footwork through the dark times, and my journal helped.

In certain groups, people who knew of my situation assured me that it was normal to be depressed. I concurred that at some point in cancer recovery (as in the grieving process), depression is a necessary stage. But, to acknowledge a never-ending burden for the rest of my life, didn't seem right. And it still doesn't. That approach is not in keeping with the *treatable and beatable* mindset that I'm hoping to convey to you.

I was so amazed that cancer had claimed me; I thought perhaps God was handing me a new life strategy. I needed to slow down, settle down, and just hang out and heal—in order to perceive what was happening. As I have said before, cancer is a wake-up call on speed dial. In deciding to fight it and hang in there, you will become stronger than you ever thought possible. Here, again, is where the mind is a powerful ally. If you want to feel like damaged goods when you are diagnosed, you have that choice. However, if you get tired of this approach and decide you feel worthy of good health and a second chance really to live this thing called life, now is the time to get on with it.

You will know you are entering the falling phase of cancer recovery when you find yourself questioning many things. Don't be afraid of these questions or answers. Just hold on to your hat and know that on the other side of this experience there is something good ahead. I'll share with you some of the questions and concerns I had:

- *Why* did this happen to me?
- What am I supposed to do when I don't feel well?
- How much activity can I truly do and still heal?
- How am I to function when my brain is affected by medications?
- When will I be able to go back to work?
- Is my work too stressful?
- Is my *life* too stressful?
- Are all my relationships healthy ones?
- If not, which ones should I reconsider?
- Is crying helpful or harmful to my immune system?
- Will my emotions ever get back to normal?
- Will I ever focus on anything besides cancer for the rest of my life?

A Rude Awakening

I wanted to use my time in the pit of despair wisely, to examine my specific areas of stress and gain some insight into how to correct or modify them. Life is full of challenges and unexpected twists, but we have the capacity to become great adapters. When I let myself fall completely, I was forced to reach out to breast cancer support groups where I sought wisdom from women who would understand the depression I was working through.

My first phone call to the American Cancer Society (ACS) was a rude awakening. Here I was in a vulnerable state, seeking support, and the people at ACS wanted me to complete a survey over the phone.

Before the voice on the phone would divulge the locations of support groups in my area, he insisted on acquiring my personal information. He ran through a list of questions involving my type of cancer, date of birth, physician, and where I was being treated. I began to feel as if I were filling out a credit application or fending off an annoying telemarketer. But because I was so eager to talk to breast cancer survivors, I endured the survey, which, after the final barrage of questions, left me feeling pretty traumatized. Why did I have to reveal private details to a stranger in order to get some simple information on support groups? I did refuse to answer a few question, such as, where was I being treated?

When I was finally given the group information, I was asked if I'd like my name placed in an outreach program, where I'd receive calls from cancer survivors. I said yes, and two messages were left on my voice mail within a few days. The first outreach call was from a woman named Rosie, a friendly voice on the phone and my first contact with the program. But, instead of offering hope and support, Rosie, too, began asking the exact questions I had refused to answer when I called the American Cancer Society. I finally asked, "Did ACS tell you to get this information from me?" She seemed surprised that I'd confronted her but abandoned the questions and proceeded to tell me her story.

The Right Kind of Support Group

I arrived at my first breast cancer support group not knowing what to expect. The first time is the hardest, of course. I sat in this small group of women, led by a facilitator who hadn't experienced the disease herself. Because I was the new kid, they asked me to begin the meeting by sharing my experiences. Since my treatment program was different from the standard, I was a bit hesitant. But I spoke honestly and from my heart. The women in the group were curious because I had avoided surgery. They asked specific questions about my chemotherapy, some of which I couldn't answer. They looked at me strangely when I didn't know the precise name and number of the chemotherapy Dr. Rubio had administered.

Here is where I trusted my doctor. He knew I was so terrified of chemo that he slipped it into my IV without my knowing. He was honoring the mind-body connection and hoped to spare me unnecessary stress. When I explained that I hadn't lost my hair as a result of my treatment, the facilitator looked at me and remarked, "You are strange!" I was taken aback by the remark. This was the comment of a paid professional, mind you, not the other survivors. Refusing to be intimidated, my quick response was, "Strange is good in my world!" It was an awkward moment, to say the least.

The other women in the group were lovely. One twenty-year survivor gave me a great deal of encouragement—just what I had come for. In spite of her kindness, I wanted to seek out a support group with a more holistic approach to treatment. All these women were talking about their cycles of chemo, their surgeries, and how their hair had changed texture when it finally grew back. They seemed to be addressing mostly the physical issues. My focus was to use this crisis to develop a greater sense of self-awareness, and to explore new principles of wellness that would enhance my life. If you want support in this way, visit www.treatableandbeatable.com for information on *Treatable and Beatable* cancer healing events, retreats, articles, teleconferences, and more.

More Bumps in the Road

About three months into my treatment, I had to deal with more than depression. I experienced an allergic reaction to my medications and had my worst week, physically speaking. During this falling phase I experienced a complete sense of physical powerlessness. When your body temperature goes from frigid to feverish, you have no choice but to ride it out. This is when I was so emotionally challenged that even my closest relationships seemed empty. I felt that no one understood, except *maybe*, the women in the support group. Okay, so focusing on the physical issues isn't a waste of time, but I am always searching for more.

One of the great encouragements the American Cancer Society support group offered me was this: You *will* get your life back...you *will* get your energy back. Most people don't like to waste time and energy. When we're healing from cancer, we need to conserve every ounce of energy we have. It's our most precious resource and determines what we can or cannot do.

Hate Hurts the Hater

The more my body was out of alignment from the medications, the more my emotions were tested. I was far from the way I wanted to be (calm and serene). Instead, I had angry bouts where I pushed people away. I didn't always express it outwardly, but my mind wielded a sword of vengeance when I thought about those who had apparently disappeared during my time of need. This is not a good way to live; hate hurts the hater.

For many years before my diagnosis, I'd felt that cancer might stem from a foundation of unresolved anger. In my mind, the "dark hole" was the storage place of these phantoms, past and present. Crawling into that hole meant facing these toxic resentments one more time. Resentment eats away at us; it's a bit like ingesting poison yourself and then hoping your enemies will die.

Healthy People Can't Fully Understand

Treatments like chemotherapy are used to treat immune system diseases other than cancer. I heard about a couple different cases where women with an overactive immune system had to take chemotherapy treatments to kill these over-stimulated cells. One gal named Angie had a story that really shed light on how emotionally fragile we are after extensive treatment.

Angie was part of a city-based book club for a number of years. When her chemotherapy treatment started, she experienced hair loss. In her case the hair loss was permanent, so one of her side effects from treatment was alopecia. Between the emotional reeling from the treatment itself, combined with the side effect of permanent hair loss, everyone in the book club quickly knew the trauma that was happening.

Angie, a pleasant literary buff, became insistent and demanding. She expressed her unrealistic expectations to the group: "Now that I'm in treatment, I think the book club should accommodate me and move the meeting location to my home in the suburbs." No one in the group knew how to handle the situation. The book club in existence for over five years had always been city-based, right in the heart of downtown Chicago. Most of the ladies lived in the city, relied on public transportation, and didn't even own cars. The neediness and demands of this chemically-altered friend basically alienated her from everyone. Fortunately, this was temporary because her story has a happy ending, and after her treatment and adjustment to alopecia, she got back together with everyone and found a wonderful new man to celebrate life with.

The First Year Journal to Review Your Emotional and Physical Process

Just like Angie, making unnecessary demands because of her own emotionally disrupted reality, it's nice to have a place to put down your highs and lows as you journey your way through treatment. A journal gives a reference record for those times when we feel we are backsliding and then suddenly discover we've gotten stronger and restored. Treatment-induced irrational behavior can happen from allergic reactions to medications and prolonged treatment side effects. Just remember that mental and moral conditioning is needed here. Spending time criticizing others or being envious of the healthy ones only hurts you. You may not recognize this irrational behavior, because the process of treatment has you so consumed, but others will. At least that is how it was for me.

Here is a thumbnail sketch of my first year of treatment. Particularly if you are going through immunotherapy or considering non-surgical options I offer this to you. By looking back on my journal, I found that each month of treatment was like a new adventure. Keeping track of my process and progress, I'll briefly share some highs and lows with you, so you don't feel so alone. Here is an abbreviated version of my roller coaster ride through the first year of treatment.

MONTH ONE

I had only one goal: staying alive and getting through each new day. My normally active lifestyle consisted of minimal exercise. Since three weeks were spent at Dr. Rubio's hospital, I made use of the pool with a little swimming, which was the best I could do. This movement helped stimulate the lymph system, so if was part of treatment, and it helped. When I finally ventured out on walks, I realized how tired I was.

MONTH TWO

Back at home, I began adjusting to a new lifestyle with the home program and all the supplements, IVs, and injections that my husband Bryan kept helping me with. I nicknamed him "Dr. Love," as his special care kept me on track. I attempted to do my exercise classes but noticed that, even in a simple routine stretch class, my body now felt stiff and old. At that point, I was probably functioning at twenty-five percent of my former capacity.

MONTH THREE

At ninety days of treatment, emotional issues began to surface. I'd gotten used to my home care program, which also included freshly-made daily juices and hot mineral salt baths each night to help detoxify the radiation and chemotherapy. With all the rituals and homework involved in my health regime, it began to feel like a full-time job. This is where the onset of depressive, dark times commenced.

MONTH FOUR

I was experiencing some serious depression. I needed more sleep than ever before. My only exercise was walking and minimal yoga; I also did a little swimming, but when I made it to any of the above activities, I was dragging myself to them. All my energy reserves seemed to be consumed by the fancy footwork, dancing with the dark times. The whole ordeal with insurance company claims was exhausting me. Certain family members just evaporated, after lending great support.

MONTH FIVE

Dr. Love, a.k.a. my husband—strikes again! He saw that I needed a change of scenery, and he took me on vacation to Hawaii. We regularly visit the islands, yet this trip was extra special. I swam with the dolphins off the coast of the Big Island of Hawaii—talk about a pinnacle healing experience—this made me feel alive again. It was the beginning of hope. I began to exercise in the gym and looked forward to healthy meal preparations. Basking in the sun seemed to recharge my battery. Sunlight, by the way, is good for healing tumors, perhaps because it's a source of vitamin D. Most importantly, I began to regain my optimism for living. I credit my husband, the dolphins, and Hawaii for all this!

MONTH SIX

After reviewing my blood work, Dr. Rubio told me that my cancer was in remission. Knowing that remission is not a synonym for cure, I said, "I want an all-clear!" He told me not quite yet. But in spite of his cautious approach, I found myself wanting to do more than my energy would allow (by now, you shouldn't be surprised). However, there were still more lessons in patience to learn. Some weeks I'd exercise more than others, keeping up with my daily juices, mineral baths, and health-building protocol was still a full-time focus. I did pop my head out of my shell and took on a few speaking engagements; it was heaven to me.

MONTH SEVEN

I really began to feel much better and took on more work projects, including this book. I felt so grateful about the treatment I'd received, and although each day had its challenges, I was also experiencing glimpses of a new life ahead. If you are newly involved in treatment, hold on to hope that there is a *month seven* to look forward to, where you start to feel like you may have cancer, but cancer doesn't have you.

MONTH EIGHT

Still impatient with my energy levels, I was acknowledging what I could and couldn't do. There were times when I'd feel so good I would overdo it, and then I would *not* feel good. I felt like a beginner learning life balance. Here was Dr. Rubio's welcomed explanation, "You are like a battery trying to get a charge. Your body has been exhausted from a big fight that drained all your battery's energy. Now you need to focus on getting your battery fully recharged." Translated, this meant more down time.

MONTH NINE

I experienced more impatience and depression. I was so tired of being out of the mainstream of life. And the careful attention to diet and all the pills started to seem like just too much work. *Did I really have any idea, when I signed on to heal cancer without surgery, how long it would take and how much work it would entail?* I'd constantly have to remind myself of my miracle; I healed stage three breast cancer without any surgery. Going from self-pity to gratitude is always a way of making progress, but after nine months I was doing more pity than thanks.

MONTH TEN

I was now doing sixty percent of the activity I'd once done, and I was frustrated. *Will this lesson in patience ever be over*, I wondered? *Will I ever be a joyful overachiever again*? I battled to adjust to what my capacities were and was scared to look into the future as to what they would eventually be. How is that for a *treatable and beatable spirit*? But on the upside, I was exercising and getting physically stronger in the gym. I felt like a corralled stallion, but I was doing my best to wait out the recuperation phase. Being a woman who questions everything, a hormone blocking pill was making my body very uncomfortable and stiff. I asked Dr. Rubio if I could get off it. He adjusted the dosage, and my energy, mood, and bloating all started to shift in a positive direction.

I have listened to many women complain about this part of the treatment (my sister-in-law calls it the yucky pill), and I encourage you to talk with your doctors to express complaints or concerns.

MONTH ELEVEN

After telling Dr. Rubio about my up-and-down energy levels, we agreed that my body needed a total detoxification process. I spent a week at the hospital with lots of IVs, fasting with fresh juices, broths, waters, and cleansing protocols. This was again more natural healing work, but it was a substantial turning point. You do know that you can be depressed from too many toxins in your body? I found my depression receding and my energy returning once I did a week-long fast. I knew I had turned a corner. I highly recommend that any patients who have good blood work investigate a detoxification program after the drug therapy is over. This is a substantial way to reclaim your vitality and health. See Chapter Nine and Resources for additional assistance.

MONTH TWELVE

My progress was evident. The bloating from the treatment finally started to leave my face and body. The first place I noticed this was my face. The body heals, top to bottom, inside to outside. Every day I was less stiff, and exercise was becoming easier. The best part of all—I finally got the coveted "cancer free" sign from Dr. Rubio, making me one happy girl! I got out in front of audiences with new stories to tell, feeling connected to audiences now more than ever before.

I chose to look at the fires in my life as the heat needed to forge precious metals. Cancer was retooling me, as if I were an emerald evolving. As I began to address the physical, psychological, and emotional roller coaster ride, my falling phase continued through the duration of my first year. For me, cancer wasn't a process I could zip into and out of. There are probably parts of it that will be with me the rest of my life.

Today I have insights and compassion I never had before. The way I was living my life, prior to this wake-up call, was to prioritize for results, achievement, and success. However, now having been through the fires of cancer, I'm more interested in expressing myself in the world, not from an egocentric focus, but from an internal passion. Suddenly, the message I would deliver to people became more important than how many top-rated conferences I had on my calendar. Offering people a road map to healthy survivorship and new options to cancer recovery became my new purpose in life.

A Battle Lost

Around the time of my remission, I heard from a friend whose husband Raul had been diagnosed with colon cancer just six months after their wedding. The doctors advised removal of part of his colon to keep the cancer from spreading. He agreed to the surgery, kept a positive attitude, and engaged in the recovery process. Soon after the first surgery, when it seemed that he was clear, my friend Keri became pregnant. The cancer didn't give up easily, and two more colon and rectum surgeries were performed. They had a thirtieth birthday cancer free celebration and new baby arrival party. This cute couple was the picture of true love, both athletic and fit people who seemed so full of life.

They hoped and believed their lives were back to normal. However, Raul's three surgeries didn't prevent the cancer from spreading. His lungs were the site of the next recurrence. Because the cancer had completely metastasized in his lungs, he went on to massive doses of chemotherapy. Eventually the cancer spread to Raul's brain, and a surgeon removed the tumor from his brain. He kept bouncing back and forth from the hospital to home because he didn't want hospice to come in. When he finally did accept that he needed hospice, he had only a short time left.

My friend Keri, the strongest wife you can imagine, called me when the end was near. I told her I'd pray for them every day. A week later, I planned to mail a greeting card on my way to the desert for another writing retreat. I called because I needed their address. When Keri answered the phone, immediately I knew that something was not right.

Raul had passed away the night before. He died three-and-a-half years after his initial cancer diagnosis; he was thirty-one years old.

As you can imagine, any cancer death, when you are still fighting for your life, is a major blow. I asked my friend if I could stop by that day on my way to the desert. What I gained from that sad visit was overwhelming gratitude for Dr. Rubio and his medicine of the future. I felt strongly that her husband's multiple surgeries had ultimately shortened his life. Had he been given some other options, he might have had at least a few more years to enjoy his family. After his death, I became even more inspired to spread the message of claiming your power when it comes to choosing a cancer treatment.

Learning to Fall so You Can Progress

If you want to feel more passion for living than you've ever felt before, I suggest you learn to fall. The hardest parts of the healing process are where the true gems reside.

Get a cancer journal now, and if you're interested in the companion journal to this book, contact the publisher. Some people wonder what to write; here are some suggestions. You can answer all the thought-provoking questions provided in this chapter, do daily or weekly entries on what your mood is, how your energy is holding up, what have been the joys and sorrows around you. It's important to document the realizations you're experiencing, in order to build yourself a new life. Please hear me: I don't know how long this new life of yours or mine will last, but I wish it to be the fullest, richest life possible.

Whether you've been a Pollyanna or a Super Stoic with a grin glued to your face, it's time to do some investigating. Here are some questions to help you chart your progress on the subject of learning to fall. I suggest you write down your answers. When you are really getting the baggage out, you'll likely feel compelled to write. But if you become bored or tired, put the pen down and wait until you're more inspired. If you're not a natural write-my-feelings-down type, here are some questions to help you get started.

THOUGHT-PROVOKING QUESTIONS

- Why do I think this has happened to me?
- What are the major frustrations in my life right now?
- What do I fear the most?
- On whom do I depend emotionally?
- What types of situations make me feel insecure?
- Am I comfortable expressing my most vulnerable feelings?
- Am I attuned to the emotional growth in my life?
- What do I love consistently, each day in my life?
- *Whom* do I love consistently, each day in my life?
- To what extent do I fully put myself out there each day? (No one can honestly claim one hundred percent.)
- In what areas am I holding back?
- What am I keeping myself from saying and to whom? Why?
- What am I keeping myself from *doing*? Why?
- What emotional issues stemming from unfinished relationships do I need to deal with now? Later?
- What crutches do I use to get through the day?
- Have I attempted to address these crutches or cravings in the past?
- Am I feeling ready now?
- Is my need to be loved satisfied?
- Is my need to be *needed* satisfied?
- Which of my passions generate more love in me each day?

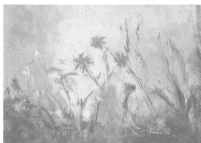

CHAPTER 7

Quelling the Emotional Storms

S cott Hamilton, the champion figure skater, has become well known for his recovery from both testicular cancer and a recent brain tumor. What I love about Scott is his *treatable and beatable* approach to cancer. He has obvious clarity about what a diagnosis has the potential to offer. In an interview he stated, "After beating cancer the first time, my awareness about life was ratcheted up. When I was diagnosed with the brain tumor this happened again, going to the next level of understanding that life is truly a gift."

Only people who have faced severe trauma or illness can understand how this ratcheting up occurs. It happens when we fully face our dire situation and decide to fight with all our might to overcome it. Once we're firmly committed, we rise to the next level of awareness and strength by riding and quelling the emotional storms.

For most of us, cancer recovery and healing are a roller coaster ride beyond compare. The word "cancer" itself automatically conjures up insecurity and fear. We have to be brave, yet vulnerable and human too. The treatment process can be grueling, and as we heal, we encounter that fine line between life and death. The drugs alone change your reality, followed by the separation from life as you knew it. Instead of going to work at 9:00 A.M., you find yourself headed for a chemotherapy treatment or another dose of radiation. These treatments trigger emotions both new and old, and when you're exhausted, they can generate emotions that run wild.

People who have never experienced serious illness are unfamiliar with the cancer terrain where patients face racing thoughts like: *How long will I live? Is the cancer gone for certain? If the cancer is truly gone, then why don't I feel better? Will I ever have my energy back and feel consistently good again?*

Some people might be able to survive this emotional terrain on their own, but if this is not your normal coping style, I suggest that you have the courage to let people in and let them see what life has done to you. I also recommend that cancer patients experience their pain and tears by asking, *What am I getting from this? What goodness is coming to me from experiencing this grief completely?* An expert in grief work, Judith Larkin Reno, Ph.D., once told me that the function of grief—if you have the courage to ride it all the way to nature's completion—is to create a new identity.

Emotional Storms from Doctors' Words

When my sister-in-law was going through breast cancer treatment, her program included a lumpectomy, followed by chemotherapy and radiation. She told her doctors that she had headaches and nausea after nine sessions of radiation. The doctors frantically said, "We need to do a brain scan to check and see if you have any brain tumors." She was petrified to say the least. Once they did the scan, they found nothing. Some of you reading this may say *that is just good medicine.* What I wonder is, based on her doctors' immediate reaction, will she now think she has a brain tumor every time she has a headache? I'd briefly like to address the impact of these types of messages given to us by medical professionals and well-wishing strangers. Some people are more sensitive than others, and treatment makes us vulnerable, when it comes to casual remarks or slips of the tongue. See if you can discipline yourself, in consideration of a patient's frail situation.

Sundays I attend my regular yoga class. One of the regulars is an advanced student named Michael. He frequently used to ask me questions about the book and the research I was doing because his mother had just been diagnosed with breast cancer. This gave him a personal interest in my treatment progress.

At the end of class one day he told another yoga student about me. Here is how he introduced me that day: "Carolyn is spearheading a campaign to give breast cancer patients options to the typical surgery method of treatment." I said, "Actually, just a campaign to give all cancer patients the message to claim their power the moment they are diagnosed and take responsibility to explore their options." Just as the words left my mouth, Michael interjected, "I forgot to tell you, Ana is a medical doctor." I said, "Oh, I see." Michael continued, "Carolyn elected to go to Mexico to get the cancer vaccine." On this pleasant Sunday morning Dr. Ana informed me, "I knew a breast cancer patient who did the same thing as you. She went to Mexico and got the cancer vaccine. Her tumors were contained for about five years, and then the cancer exploded in her body. She just had a mastectomy and is now undergoing chemotherapy."

That was quite a message to take in, when you're in a completely relaxed frame of mind. I didn't see it coming, but once the remark landed it was a familiar feeling of "being hit by a cannon ball," like my prior experiences at the surgeon's office and my "visit" with the liver specialist. Now I can add a female to my list of doctors who offer scare tactics instead of encouragement.

How difficult would it have been for Dr. Ana to keep the story of the woman with the exploding cancer to herself? I look back and think she was probably relaxed, too, and it just slipped out. What I would have preferred was a supportive remark stating, *You're cancer free—that is great!* When I look at people who feel obligated to tell a gloom-and-doom story, I assume these people tell their scary stories because either they are medically trained this way or they are scared themselves. The hardest part of the whole ordeal was that her remark left an undercurrent for emotional storms. One more doctor essentially saying, *I don't believe you've solved your problem.*

But instead of focusing on that, my next thought was about the cancer patient Dr. Ana had described. I wondered whether this patient took the road of life-enhancing cancer? Did she take time out and gain the lessons of learning to fall? Did she attack the cancer with the processes I've discussed? Did she delve into the deeper layers of the healing process, or was she running scared the entire time, attempting to outrun the cancer?

As I advocate the *treatable and beatable* mindset to life and healing without surgery, I do know that my future may not be any type of *cancer-free certainty*. What I do believe in is all my choices so far, and I will continue to believe in the choices I've made for the rest of my days. See, cancer has made me both stronger and smarter. I wonder how many patients Dr. Ana knows who can say that...I hope many. I make this bold statement because Dr. Rubio's treatment program helps with making his patients smarter. With a more holistic approach and less evasive treatment, you get less damage to the cells, including brain and memory cells. We also get stronger when we claim our power right at the beginning of the treatment.

From Self-Reliance to Self-Acceptance to Self-Possession

It is so important during treatment to understand the cycles of nature and to allow time for the emotional process to become real. On a return flight from a business trip to Costa Rica, someone left a copy of the *New Yorker* magazine in my seat pocket. In it I found an article about a prima ballerina and how her adversities changed her into becoming an exceptional performer. Her story illustrates the importance of quelling emotional storms as part of gaining greater self-awareness when we move through life's challenges.

Wendy Whelan is considered one of the greatest ballerinas of her time. She has been with the New York City ballet for twenty years. In her youth, Ms. Whelan was actually considered too thin to become a ballerina. She also questioned whether she was pretty enough for her profession, with her Corcoran nose, skinny racehorse legs, long willowy arms, and short-waist torso. She even had a curved spine in her youth that put her in a body cast. One critic reported, "She looked like a famine victim on stage." Shaken by a lack of confidence, she went through rough patches in her late twenties with failed relationships, and solicited support from her parents who were mired in their own difficulties.

It was then that Ms. Whelan realized she had to learn to "stand on her own two feet," a cliché that takes on new meaning when coming from a prima ballerina. She reflected upon her growth through emotional storms as the *tough and tricky steps from self-reliance to self-acceptance to self-possession.* Bravo to all those of you who are ready to dance your way through this process—the essence of this book is in this one phrase. Here is a quote by Mikhail Baryshnikov describing Ms. Whelan's talent, "She's the best, there's a complexity, a sense of internal life. You're always trying to decode this person when she moves."

Quelling the emotional storms in our lives, allowing them to surface, and then moving on, is how we go from self-reliance to self-possession. Later in her career, after this profound realization, Ms. Whelan had still more emotional storms to conquer. During a City Ballet trip to Russia, she went up on her toes on an unfamiliar stage while dancing in the Bolshoi Ballet Theater, and tore plantar fascia tissue in her left foot. This injury left her leg in a cast, and she lay immobilized for four months. In her words, "This hiatus completely rearranged the way I saw the world, 180 degrees."

Although her dance artistry had always been brilliant, when Ms. Whelan returned to the stage after this injury, she had a new sense of freedom and joy that was clearly translated into her performances. Chip Brown, in his *New Yorker* article, wrote, "Wendy can clearly take your breath away and you don't know why." Her choreographer added, "You don't understand why watching a leg unfold can speak volumes and how she can make you feel there is something inexpressibly beautiful about it." I know her story gives me courage to keep finding those places where I've demonstrated self-reliance and surrendered to self-acceptance, so I can be a better poised person when it come to self-possession.

Where are you right now in your dance from reliance to acceptance to possession? Generally speaking, people don't allow their emotional storms to surface. We are taught early on to believe that *only babies cry, we should keep a stiff upper lip, and hold our head high*. Yet having the courage to cycle through your emotional evolvement can hold many a treasure for those who dare to engage fully in this dance.

Facing Adversity

Some of us are born into major storms, such as the late, great Ray Charles. He was born with sight, but at the age of six months, his father walked out, leaving Ray and his mother living in such poverty that he would later say, "There was nothin' below us 'cept the ground." At five he saw his younger brother drown, and soon after he developed such severe glaucoma that by age seven, he was totally blind. Ray's mother, who died eight years later, told her son, "You might not be able to do things like a person who can see, but there are always two ways to do everything. You've just got to find the other way."

Our entire life, before, during, and after cancer, is based on our belief systems about this disease. My belief is that you must face the adversity head on, which is a factor in self-reliance. You have to love yourself through your tears, depression, anger, and ugly times, which equates to self-acceptance. And if you have the courage to do steps one and two, you will arrive at self-possession. This is what Scott Hamilton and Wendy Whelan embody. They both have some profound answers to life challenges; this gives them stability and watch-ability, with fans anticipating their next move.

Some people think that after cancer, *I'll never be the same*. I remember one colleague telling me, "You are living through my worst nightmare." Emotional storms can be a strange ride because we often don't know when they are going to surface, and we can find ourselves in the middle of some strange emotional configurations. Please heed my warning: If you are going through hell...don't stop! Just keep right on going, and you'll ride it out. There is a popular country song with these lyrics: Play it loud if you need to.

Riding the Memory Train

During my early months of treatment a friend gifted me with a *watsu* massage, which is done in a warm pool with the body stretched into various positions while floating. The massage therapist was an older man, very gentle and loving. As he worked on my body, I felt waves of panic, as I unexpectedly experienced a spontaneous age regression.

By allowing the emotional storms to surface in my body, I was experiencing the cleansing of a childhood wound. Releases of grief are like being disassembled, because a new life is being constructed from the pain. During and even after months of treatment, I felt vulnerable and infantile, much like a little tot trying to cross a street at rush hour.

Memory is active throughout our lives. Conclusions and assessments are made and stored in the subconscious. Some are pleasant, others profound. Some are dark and toxic. Those are the ones with the greatest possibility for bringing about change. If unpleasant memories are running your life, there is a need for healing.

Life-altering crises have this power to transform us, whether they involve illness, accidents, or loss of property or position. We can cycle up in crisis. We can find a way to be more.

As memories surfaced, I intended to address and clear out old baggage to be free once more. Often during sleep, I'd revisit stages of my life, as if my past were flashing before my eyes.

One night while riding the memory train, I re-lived my father's tragic accident. We were on a Christmas holiday in Puerto Vallarta when he met with a wave that changed his life. While we were bodysurfing, a rouge wave came up and propelled my six-foot father head first into the sand, snapping the vertebrae in his neck. Like Christopher Reeves, my father was instantly paralyzed. That night, as I relived my father's accident, I revisited the helpless feeling of calling out for help on the beach—to God and everyone else around. It had been a heartrending but heroic event for me, since I was the one who brought him to shore where doctors and nurses resuscitated him back to life. For the first time in ten years I experienced only the tragic part, and I allowed my heroic actions to slip aside. That single event propelled me forward with the courage to quit my secure sales job and go for my dream, doing the work I love today.

When I was in the hospital, I rode the emotional wave of my dad's demise. The tears of sadness I released had been in my heart for a decade. For all these years after the loss of my dad, I kept focusing on the transformation this experience had provided, but I never let myself fully grieve. That is the word: *fully*. Sometimes the emotional storms we process during cancer are events of the past, events we already have dealt with. Don't be surprised if you have to heal these fully one more time. I even had a shaman medicine woman tell me candidly right before my cancer treatment, "Connect more with your emotions. Your emotions are the compass. You have shut down some part of you that lets these emotions flow. Allow yourself to have more time to experience and express all your feelings."

Fully Express Your Feelings

When you finally allow yourself to connect fully with your emotions, you will suddenly feel lighter. I experienced the healer's wisdom firsthand, especially after I explored the memories of my father from a new vantage point of loss and tragedy.

Memory is always active, day and night. There were often nights I'd dream of old boyfriends, old girlfriends. I'd think about my elementary, high school, and college years without consciously conjuring up these memories. Another friend once told me she compared the subconscious mind with the mud pots in Yellowstone. Here the earth proudly displays its own bubbling up activity. Geysers and vents, where hot water and air are being released, display the Earth is very active at its core, just like we are!

So many people never touch base with this core or raw emotion until they are thrown into a battle for their lives in an emotionally charged situation, where you can't hide out in *busy-ness*. This is when many are forced to face feelings and facts. It takes courage to let the emotional storms roll and to ride the memory train. But the sky gets clearer each time we face the dark clouds that have shadowed our lives at one time or another.

Editing Toxic Memories

One Memorial Day Sunday I found myself unusually emotional during a church service, as we remembered those who had sacrificed their lives to protect our freedom. It was the Reverend Brian's birthday, and he raised the roof with his poignant message. He talked about re-membrance and shared a story about being taken advantage of when lending money. Because he was speaking from his core, he triggered memories from *my* life, and there I was, riding the memory train once more.

The story about lending money reminded me of an incident twenty years earlier when I was befriended by two men who lived next door. During this period I inherited a little money from my grandmother. Although nobody knew of my good fortune, almost the day I depos-ited the check, my next-door neighbor asked if I could loan him $1,000 for the rent. He said, "I'll pay you at the end of the week." When the time to collect arrived, he gave me only $200. After several attempts to retrieve the balance, I never received another cent. Only later did I real-ize that one of the men had a gambling problem.

After this incident, each day was a daily discomfort I had to face. In order to get to my condo, I had to walk by my neighbors. Sometimes the guys would look up from their kitchen window and smirk as I passed by. The incident planted in my mind a memory message that needed editing, "I am easily taken advantage of and misled."

That was the memory that came to me this memorial weekend, a remembrance I needed to heal. There were so many other messages I could have had from this incident; instead, this event was an emotional storm swirling with a memory message saying, "You are such a fool, easily mislead and taken advantage of." That Sunday morning after

Reverend Brian's sermon, I decided to correct and edit this memory message.

First, I gave myself credit for the display of generosity and trust in my act of lending money, when I had money to lend. Never did my mind give me credit for this.

Usually, in any situation where we feel foolish and misled, there is likely an act of courage that goes unnoticed by us. The editing process was me acknowledging my courageous act and planting a revised message that accentuates the positive. In this example, the new thought was, *People see me as a wise, powerful, resourceful person,* or making this an affirmation: *I am a generous, wise, powerful, resourceful person who wants to help others.* When you get the right edit, it clearly makes more sense and reflects a world of difference.

I'm talking about detective work when I advise people to edit their toxic memories as part of the emotional healing process. Find the stories that have delivered a painful message that is haunting you and allow yourself to heal the shame or guilt. A good detective can always find the courage you displayed in the situation or strength you gained and edit the hurtful message with something that reflects the glory, not the blame. When you get the new message in place, it clicks as the truth for your world now.

The Ride of a Lifetime

You can take a crisis like cancer—or any trauma—and make it the ride of your life. As you travel through these emotional storms in recovery, pretend you're Sherlock Holmes, and engage in this suggested detective work. Don't resist painful and emotional memories. Allow the pinnacle memory messages to surface and edit them. This experience will change your world and open your future to better possibilities.

After revisiting my memory of lending money, I gained a whole new perspective. I realized that because of a mere $800, I never lent money again! I definitely put up a shield of protection after this experience, so in actuality it was a pretty cheap lesson.

Why do these toxic memories with invaluable lessons take so much time and energy? It's because they reside at the cellular level. We can't release them until they come bubbling up from the subconscious, which is why this process is so mysterious and profound. You have to let go of your illusion of control and yield to a higher healing force. When you start trusting your life and affirming your power in all situations, the subconscious mind will do its clearing in perfect order.

For me, memories don't revel themselves in a chronological order, for they are part of a larger process. The money lending lesson came up during this sermon where I was experiencing a familiar discomfort. With my insurance not paying for my medical claims, I felt like I was being taken advantage of. It was as though I'd arrived at a station on the memory train titled "Being Taken Advantage Of" and was being asked to explore all those situations in my life that fit. Then, when my memory messages were "edited," I could resume my journey and move on.

Treatment Triggers Emotions That Need to Heal

There are logic-based people and emotion-based ones. Logic-based people will have more contemplation and reflection compared to the emotional types with Kleenex and catharsis. Since I'm the latter, before each treatment I would naturally experience both fears and tears. Perhaps I was crying because I was not well and had to endure these inoculations? All I know is that I needed to clear my emotional landscape to prepare for what was coming. All the emotional storms and editing toxic memories would actually focus me in the physical fight for my life. Since I had no idea what exact symptoms I'd experience from each different vaccine, crying was a release that strengthened me.

The same is true with chemotherapy and radiation. Before any of these treatments, you can get those tears and fears out. And after the treatments, it is wise to protect oneself because the body is engaged in its own physical crisis. When each treatment battle ends, the rewards can be great, with often a renewed strength of hope and purpose.

I don't think anyone really wants to deal with emotional storms. I resisted delving into the past, where emotions that were too tough to handle at the time had been stored in my body. Clearing emotional baggage is a lot like cleaning out a closet. If we can't decide what to do with a certain item, we tend to stuff it into a closet, and we might not open that closet for months, years, or ever.

Do You Need a Retreat to Quell the Emotional Storms?

If you are having difficulty doing this type of emotional or logical clearing at home (and are well enough), I suggest you go on a solitary retreat for a minimum of three nights or more. Visit a favorite place, away from people and chaos, where natural beauty is easy to access. Get yourself to a place near water, the mountains, the desert, a favorite rural area or some natural wonder. Pack up your medicines and special foods so there will be no interruption in your health routine. Find a place that inspires you, perhaps a place where you've always wanted to go. Now you finally have some time, so spend it wisely.

Take along a journal, uplifting or inspiring music you love, healthy snacks, and walking shoes. Plan to sleep well, and if possible walk around and experience your new environment. As you move outside your familiar arena, see what memories are playing out; notice if there is a haunting feeling about someone or something in the past that is unresolved. Instead of stuffing it back in the closet, coax it out. In an interview actor Tom Hanks said, "We must constantly be examining who we are, how we got here, and how we are getting through all this."

Be an adventurer as you travel the terrain of emotional storms. These emotions can be triggered by medical procedures, frustrations, insensitive people, or the loss of your former life as you knew it. This exploration is so important to the healing process because carrying around the emotional baggage of unresolved anger and grief creates more stress and burdens the immune system. It also prevents you from seeing the blessings you've had in your life. I think there is real freedom when we allow a *cancer cleaning of our emotional closets* and discard the baggage. When tears are near the surface, get them out.

There are times with the bigger emotion-packed memories when they are on their way to clear that you may feel disoriented—possibly ill or just flat crazy. May I suggest that knowledge is power; wait before you reach for some quick-fix pill to make this process go away, especially if you sense you are really on an emotional clearing path. Ride out the storm; a new sense of freedom is on the other side.

Find a truth-telling buddy who can listen to you throughout the roller coaster ride of your treatment—someone who knows and cares. Tell that person what you are doing, and ask for his or her support. We often place spouses or relatives in this role, but someone outside your immediate circle may offer fresh insights and lift some of the burden from your caregivers and family.

If going on a retreat is absolutely a new adventure for you, and you're not sure where to start, following are some questions to stimulate thought. And if you are someone who prays, ask for guidance during your healing retreat to address those things that are holding you back in life, so you can be a stronger, healthier person once this ordeal is over. If you have never felt successful with journaling or just don't know what this "journaling thing" is all about, here are a few suggestions: Buy the *Treatable and Beatable* companion journal for this book or a special new notebook to record your cancer recovery thoughts. Maybe have a ritual where you sit down and light a candle before you start to write. Detail the day, the emotions, or thoughts you had just planning this getaway retreat. What are the outcomes you hope are ahead for you after cancer is over? Detail them. What do you want to do differently? Maybe write a letter to yourself in three years, describing how wonderful and happy you are. What would you like to see happening in your world? Perhaps there is someone you deeply miss; write them a letter and tell them how much they meant in your life. All these suggestions get us in touch with our core essence and the things that matter.

QUELLING THE EMOTIONAL STORMS JOURNALING QUESTIONS

1. What has been my predominant emotion since my diagnosis? Give a play-by-play of the way you have responded. Which parts have been hardest to manage? Where have you been strong?

2. What has been my predominant emotion this week or month? Do I know of a specific incident that triggered this emotion? Explain in detail and elaborate. Answers come when we let the pen go and flow. If it is a major emotional storm, it helps to write about it at length before proceeding to the next question.

3. Do I want to share this situation with someone so I don't have to go it alone? Can I?

4. Who are the persons who would be most supportive, understanding, and available to talk to on any issue? List your truth-telling friends. Who is the best person to talk to on this issue? Call them!

5. After I vent my emotional storm and write the play-by-play in my journal, what have I gained, what insights do I now possess that this storm has done—both *to* me and *for* me? What toxic messages need to be "edited," and how have they affected my life?

6. What gift can I give myself this week for managing my recovery process regarding this emotional event? What are the healing messages I want to put in place, now that I've reviewed these incidents once more?

7. How do I visualize my life in three years? What changes have I made, and what goals have I reached? Be very detailed about this so you can actually *see* the end result.

8. Who have been the greatest friends in my life? List them. Who have been my greatest adversaries? (I like to call these people "teachers.") To help release specific resentments, the next chapter and questions at the end will be beneficial.

CHAPTER 8

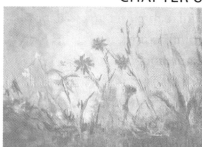

Anger Can Heal

I feel so strongly about addressing anger as a crux of healing cancer that it is the one emotion that gets an entire chapter. You don't have to be a patient to benefit from the suggestions herein. Sometimes emotional storms envelop family members who are not ill but have had their lives turned upside down by the impact of a loved one with cancer.

We need to address anger because it causes great loads of stress. And stress and healing do not complement each other.

The Impact of Anger

A woman named Toni once discussed her life story with my spiritual study group. She lived in a retirement home and complained bitterly about how bad things were. She had financial resources, was in good health, and made frequent contact with her daughter and grandchildren. Her retirement setup seemed to have all the necessary components for happiness, yet she often expressed fits of anger. She was so busy pointing fingers and complaining about everyone from her family to the other retirement home residents that the group rarely heard anything about her, other than her extensive complaints. It was interesting, as an outsider, to listen when she shared her so-called trials. Once in a while she would stop and say, "There's so much anger in me—I don't understand it."

Observing her unhappy demeanor and constant complaints made me all the more determined to face my own emotional storms, especially anger as it surfaced. Negative people can be inspiring to us, too, as they illustrate how we don't want to live.

Another gentleman was a business acquaintance who lost his mother to breast cancer when he was only six years old. In adulthood he was ambitious, earning a good dollar, yet suffered from fits of anger and depression. Even as he recalled his impressive business accomplishments, he would say, "I've got anger issues, and I get depressed frequently."

He was a brilliant businessman and sometimes a hilariously funny guy, yet there was always this anxiety within him. You could tell he never knew when he was going to lose his temper or behave strangely. One day when he revealed the details of his mother's death, I learned volumes. My observation was this man had never fully faced his painful childhood loss. His father was a military man who had encouraged him to soldier on when his mother died. I concur with the philosophy of marching ahead, but only after you have acknowledged the blow of abandonment and allowed the healing process to take place. The process of expressing and quelling these emotional storms is vital to self-possession.

When this gentleman "lost it" during his repeated angry outbursts, it seemed that his wife used his bad behavior to her gain. His anger gave her buying power. I saw firsthand how he never fully grieved his loss and was carrying this angry turmoil with him all these years.

A System to Help Heal Anger

Anger is a part of life and a natural emotion that comes up during unexpected events like cancer. In life, events occur, and we react. Once you interpret a situation as unfair, an injustice, disappointment, abandonment, violation, etc., you then progress to identify the issue and have engaged in the cycle. I'm going to explain briefly a system that can help us heal anger or at least help us comprehend how to heal anger when we are ready.

I learned about the anger cycle from Taylor Hartman, Ph.D., bestselling author of *The Color Code*. His is a powerful book about identifying your core motive in life. Because I believe in this motive concept, I want to tell you about Taylor's philosophy regarding healing anger and the anger cycle. When I first heard about this, I was going through the ordeal called cancer. I had the opportunity to experience his concepts directly and intimately on more than one occasion. What a world of difference when you directly experience something versus hearing about the concept. The insights gained are immense. Here is an overview of what Taylor Hartman talks about in the anger cycle. Start at the top and travel clockwise.

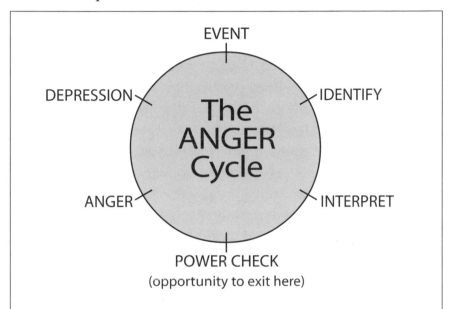

EVENT

DEPRESSION

The ANGER Cycle

IDENTIFY

ANGER

INTERPRET

POWER CHECK
(opportunity to exit here)

EVENT—Triggering event that brings forth strong feelings.

IDENTIFY—A person must identify what their feelings are, and what exactly triggered them.

INTERPRET—Next the person interprets the event for the cause-effect connection and begins to analyze what can be done.

POWER CHECK (opportunity to exit here)—The person then does a power check within himself to determine if s/he has the skills and power to resolve the situation. If the answer is yes, steps are taken to resolve it, and the anger is usually diffused.

ANGER—A heightened state of powerlessness, helplessness, or injustice. Takes a lot of energy.

DEPRESSION—Anger turned inward. Instead of being a volcano actively spewing, depression is like the live coals burning dormant inside. Three options here: (1) stay depressed, (2) jump ship, or (3) go around The Anger Cycle again.

A Few Trips Around the Anger Cycle

To illustrate how this process works, I am going to outline a couple of relationship scenarios that really shifted during my cancer recovery process. These stories aren't meant to blame or shame anyone; they are simply a part of my life, and they illustrate the power of the cancer experience and how it can be transforming. When I talk about transformation, I'm referring to correcting those personality flaws that pertain to my life.

These situations triggered deep and sudden anger in me, and using the anger cycle is how I helped process them as a catalyst in my own growth. This is what any good therapist does. Sometimes we can do this work on our own if we have the tools, skills, and support system. I hope these stories will illustrate how injustices can end up healing dormant anger and free us forever (or until the next event occurs).

I didn't anticipate these events, and when they occurred during my cancer recovery, I reacted differently than I had in the past. They all took place in the latter months of treatment, when the tumor was gone. With the physical danger of cancer at bay, my anger issues began to surface. In some ways, I think I was more reactive to any unkindness because I felt like life had already been unkind to me. In other words, I was like a volcano ready to blow or a trip wire set to detonate if I was disrupted.

An Unresponsive Relative

In the beginning of recovery, many people make a fuss, sending prayers, notes, and gifts. But often, even when cancer is in remission, most patients still have treatments to deal with. And all too frequently, as soon as you tell people that the tumor is gone, they assume the ordeal is over and all is fine. Of course, a fellow "thriver" knows better, which is why we need each other.

I had a cousin on the East Coast I kept in touch with. We were best buddies while growing up. She, in fact, was the first one I called when I discovered the tumor, partially because a few years earlier her husband had committed suicide. I knew she understood the impact of sudden devastating news. She and her daughter prayed for me and placed my name on her church prayer list. Because of all these supportive activities, it rekindled our bond, similar to what we had as children.

I was about nine months into treatment and had been feeling ill for a couple of weeks following a specific vaccine. I was vulnerable and needed extra emotional support. I called my cousin over the Fourth of July weekend, but by the end of July she still hadn't returned my call. I was disappointed, but had no idea how much anger I was accumulating as the weeks ticked by without hearing from her. She finally did return my call around mid-August and left a voicemail message. I chose not to respond. That was my way of saying, "I'm hurt so I won't return your call either." Here is how this occurrence fits into the anger cycle diagram:

The Event: I made a phone call to my cousin while I was going through cancer treatment, and she did not return my call with any sense of priority or promptness.

Identify: Her not returning my call made me question her sincerity and love when I'd offered support to her for years after her difficult situation with her husband's death.

Interpret: I deserved a return call. I was nine months into battling cancer. Expectation: I've helped you before…you owed me. Here is where the juice happened. I've had people wait to return a phone call before, but in this situation it was like waiting on the pony express. I decided I won't be waiting for her call or making any more.

Power Check: This is where I felt powerless. My own cousin wouldn't make me a priority and return my call.

Anger: I was very angry with her and in some ways with other family members who never even acknowledged I was sick.

Depression: I had anger that turned to sadness, because staying angry all the time is exhausting. I saw this cousin as a close family member. Other relatives and cousins never bothered to call. This triggered for me sadness at how much support was in my family overall.

Exiting the Anger Cycle There are two places you can exit the anger cycle; the first is the Power Check phase, the second is the Depression phase.

Power Check: If you exert your power, you can interrupt the cycle and exit here. Do we have the power to do something about this, or are we powerless? When we initiate our power we start to feel better. I'll illustrate in a moment how I did this with my cousin.

According to Taylor Hartman's theory, in the Power Check phase, if you cannot exert your own power, you can reassess the anger and exit in the depression phase. When it comes to the depression phase, you have three choices.

1) You can stay depressed with an attitude that life isn't fair and that you've been treated badly. (This was the example of Toni.) You then have this baggage you carry around for a very long time until you find a way to exit the cycle.

2) You can work your way back to anger and get back to reassessing your power. If you can find your power in the situation, often this comes from seeing what the event has done to make you grow, then you can exit.

3) You can disengage or in Taylor Hartman's words, "jump ship," and say, "I'm done with this relationship."

Here is what happened and how the situation played out. When my cousin returned my call in mid-August and left a voice mail, I did not return her call. On Labor Day weekend I placed a call to my mother's house, to say hello.

Surprise! My cousin who lives three states away was answering my mother's phone. At first I didn't recognize her voice, and when she asked,

"Is that you, Carolyn?" I responded, "Who is this?" It was then I knew it was her. I was so shocked and angry I merely repeated, "Is my mother there?" When my cousin told me, "Your Mother isn't here," I mumbled a quick thank you and hung up.

Here I was calling in the midst of a family gathering, and *bang!* I hung up on a cousin I've known all my life. That was me exerting my power and not playing nice. It shocked me really...was this really *me* being so abrupt? My behavior was based on the event that I had already identified and interpreted months earlier. I'd instinctively chosen not to deal with her that day. I didn't want to stuff my feelings with trivialities: *Oh, how nice to hear your voice—Are you having a good weekend?* So I flat out didn't.

Actions like this have a ripple effect, and since my cousin was visiting our mutual relatives, I realized that everyone would hear about my rude behavior. But did that give me second thoughts or an incentive to call back and behave differently? No. I was making a stand, asserting my power. My well-mannered-people-pleasing facade was no longer in place. I firmly believe that had I played nice that Labor Day weekend, I would have felt even more depressed and stayed in the anger cycle even longer.

Reflecting back on the situation with my cousin, I realized that the times we'd talked about my cancer ordeal, she was still fighting her own battles. As a single mom, she had a hectic life, huge responsibilities, and little energy to spare. For me to expect anything close to full-time support from her for my emotional cancer storms while living three states away was too much. So if I had interpreted this initially with more compassion, I wouldn't have had to go around the anger cycle at all. We have mended our relationship. She did apologize, and I have since realized you can't expect too much of others, even relatives.

What became clear to me in this situation is that our support systems can shift. People we thought we could count on sometimes don't make it to the finish line. The cancer battle, especially healing cancer without surgery, is a long one. There is also anger aroused by a life-threatening illness, and it will come out in the strangest ways. These stories are to offer hope, so you don't feel like you are the only one going through these things.

A Fractured Friendship

For years I had been sharing my life journey with one particular friend. She was a mental health professional, helping people, as I was with my counseling, coaching, and speaking. We were both working to improve our lives and help others. She had been there for me during the early stages of my marriage and my business. I had witnessed her putting her marriage back together after she had discovered her husband's sex addiction, raising and home schooling three children, and finally, landing her dream job.

We had been friends for over a decade when the fracture happened. She worked in Palm Desert, and we had a favorite restaurant there. I was planning a trip to the area, so I called ahead and suggested dinner one summer night. She returned my call promptly, with a voicemail saying, "Our favorite place is closed for the summer." End of message. She suggested no alternatives and added no closing phrases like "talk to you later."

At the same time I offered a dinner invitation, I was preparing for advanced training to become further certified for my seminar work. Part of the preparation involved giving five evaluations to friends, family, and employees to complete on my behalf. I requested that she do an evaluation for me, based on the years and the depth of our friendship. I tried to make the evaluations as anonymous as possible, so that people would be honest as they assessed my strengths and weaknesses.

Shortly after my friend left that cryptic message, she left another one: "I can't fill out this evaluation—I'm going to mail it back to you." She gave no further explanation. The two voicemails together had a strong impact; my jaw about hit the floor. I had no idea why she had taken a pass on dinner or why she couldn't spend twenty minutes on an evaluation after a decade long friendship. I never heard from her again.

Taking this scenario to the Anger Cycle:

Event: Long-time friend turns down dinner invitation and evaluation request. .

Identify: As a healthcare professional, she knows how these personal development processes work. It was the lack of explanation combined with the abrupt voicemails that triggered my interpretation. I felt she was abandoning the friendship, and the refusal to do the evaluation fueled disappointment or unmet expectations.

Interpret: To me at the time, her actions indicated she didn't value our friendship too much. As I looked over the past ten years, I realized this was a more or less one-sided relationship.

Power Check: She had the power in our relationship by never initiating phone calls or being together. We shared things in common, but her disclosure levels were never at a level displaying the vulnerability of true friendship.

I now no longer need people in my life who don't extend this availability and vulnerability. I decided to exit the anger cycle and jump ship, which shifted my focus from helplessness to acceptance.

With the loss of the friend, it took less time for me to process the anger and hurt. The pain and anger from this sudden rift propelled me to select friends who reciprocate friendship. Where did I get the idea that I should keep people in my life who don't appreciate me? These beliefs usually come from somewhere in your childhood and have to be healed.

The Experience of Anger Overload

With all the editing of toxic stuff, between relationship disappointments, insurance battles, and uncertainty of when I could have a normal life again, I became physically consumed with anger. Before you start to wonder about my "anger issues," let me comment that one of the stages of grief is anger. What I was experiencing with this overreacting phase in my cancer recovery was that my anger over my entire situation was blurring my reality and making me less tolerant. I also think the anger was most volatile when it was exiting my being.

One dear friend said I was "flooding" with anger. When you have anger issues exiting, you can have a "10" response on the anger scale over a minor "2" event, such as just going to the dry cleaners and finding they don't have your clothes ready when promised. At this point minor incidents let me know I was living on a volcano and putting out fires.

If I barely recognized myself when I hung up on my cousin that Labor Day weekend, this new unfamiliar rage made me a complete stranger to myself. I questioned whether I would ever be happy and have a compassionate heart again. As I look back now, I feel certain an entire lifetime of anger was releasing from me. I wish I'd had a white light experience, where it was miraculously lifted away, but instead I had to ride it out for months. I learned that this is exactly the time when it becomes imperative to *trust the process*. It finally did shift, briefly, into depression and then into a level of awareness I had never known before.

Getting Un-Screwed

If you can relate to any of these stories, let me give you some encouragement. When you set out to heal anger, each infraction becomes a vehicle of transformation. If people in your life are intentionally trying to hurt you, they are, in fact, actually making you stronger. That said, a more common scenario is that their actions are inconsiderate rather than deliberate and are also sometimes the result of battling beasts of their own.

Here is a philosophy I hold dear when I coach clients. If earlier in your life you screwed up or were "screwed," then getting healthy means you have to get *un*-screwed. When we come from environments where emotions are suppressed, abuse occurs, problems are ignored, and nurturing is in short supply, then this can be a screwed-up situation. From these unsettled experiences, your stability later in life can be shaky at best.

Let's say you figure out that you need some help with anger and want to make changes based on your decision to be healthy and present. Hold on for a ride as you start to express emotions, stop abusing yourself, address problems, and nurture yourself. This process of cycling up to a new life means you have to review your early reality before you can exit the anger cycle to live happily and productively. I call this process getting *un*screwed. Getting unscrewed is like a dance with the dark stuff. It can be difficult but profound; releasing anger is an experience that will result in greater personal power and awareness.

Anger Is One Letter Away from Danger

If we can really slow down and review our lives, we'll surely find out where the bones are buried. I have to say that when I began to inventory my relationships, I got in touch with long-buried anger. But for me this anger was healing and no less dramatic than the medical-physical-emotional fight with cancer. First, I had to heal the physical malady, and then the emotional ones became apparent.

You do know that "anger" is one letter away from "danger"? If you're spending lots of time with anger, you're also spending time in danger. The danger for a cancer patient is his own human ecosystem is poisoned by resentments. We literally can't afford these draining emotions; we need our strength and reserves for the task of restoring health.

We Need to Feel Our Feelings

Jenny was diagnosed with stage one breast cancer. Her nursing background made her savvy in her matter-of-fact approach to her diagnosis. She claimed her power by having a lumpectomy and radiation, but saying no-thank-you to chemotherapy. Yet, as she stoically went about having her successful treatment, here is what she tearfully told me one day when she was clear of cancer: "I'm afraid I'm getting depressed. I can't handle depression; I just can't. I'd rather have cancer again than feel depressed, and I can feel this depression just wanting to overtake me, but I won't give in." I suggested to her, "You may need to feel your feelings here rather than do an escape dance away from depression. Given the situation, it isn't realistic. Just allow your feelings to flow and pass through." She got it; she just needed to be reminded that depression stems from suppressed emotions (including anger); release the emotion and move on.

Another woman trying to get her health on track after cancer was dealing with an eating disorder. She spoke of her quick-fix methods to break food addiction and how she would often abandon programs that were helping her. She was angry, too. She would relate in a heated tone, "Why at seventy years old after facing cancer do I still having to deal with this eating stuff?"

After acknowledging the repressed anger and depression in my own life, I realized that many women were struggling with the same burden. Anger is a toxic emotion, much like envy and resentment. The purpose of healing anger is to lighten your load so you can live post-cancer or during cancer, without all this excess baggage. I have always felt instinctively that cancer is a disease related to repressed anger. I do not agree with those who deny the stress-cancer connection, for I truly believe there is a link. Part of my healing is to take responsibility for patterns in my personality that may have contributed to my illness.

Healing Anger from the Core Versus Lip Service

It's one thing to tell someone *I forgive you*, as we're often instructed to do in self-help books and programs. However, when we really free ourselves from resentment, it's not just lip service; it's a whole new state of mind. Anger, hostility, and resentment constrict, trap, and diminish us, but healing and forgiveness expand us and give us greater compassion. Remember Jesus saying to *love your enemies*. And that means more than just saying the words, because love is a core emotional expression.

Here are some suggestions to help you *feel your feelings* and transform yourself in the process.

MAINTAIN BALANCE WHILE EXPERIENCING AND HEALING ANGER

Bring on the Laughter: When you are inundated with rage, stop the toxicity and take a break. Go rent a comedy or watch something funny on TV. Balance the circuitry so that you don't become a raging fool. Tell yourself: *I'm through obsessing about this situation and letting this person control me.* See if you can distract yourself with laughter to offset the pain.

Kid Therapy: If you have kids in your life (or can borrow one), they, too, can be a pleasurable distraction. Spend some time talking to a two-year-old or a kindergartener. Play with him or her at home or go to the park where people are actively having fun. Bear witness to childlike innocence.

Write for Your Life: Write a letter (which you must promise never to mail) to the person(s) you resent or feel you hate. Go ahead and call them every name in the book—let it all out on paper. Be specific in listing perceived transgressions such as lying, cheating, or acts of outright cruelty. Your sentence for these injustices is to ban that person from your life.

Act It Out: If writing isn't your cup of tea, or if the written word isn't enough, engage in a little play-acting. Conjure up an image of the offending party, sit him or her down in a chair, and read that person the riot act. By releasing your pent up feelings verbally and with great emotion, you can attain a feeling of power—and release.

Shout It Out: If an Oscar-worthy performance doesn't do it for you, let your emotions out full-force—into a pillow. Scream and yell bloody murder, and hope your vocal cords will make it through. When we release unexpressed anger by finding our (full-blast) voice, we may pay with some throat sensitivity, but in the greater scheme of things, it's a small price.

Get Physical: Physical activity is another way to release the anger from your body. Do whatever you like best, whether it's tennis, gardening, or just walking. Or try something new. I discovered *dejembe*, a form of African drumming, right around the time I was releasing my anger scenarios. Pounding on a drum did more for me than a year of psychotherapy. It's also wonderful for breast cancer, because by drumming you are specifically targeting and releasing tension in the upper body. To locate African drumming circles in your neighborhood, just go online.

Healing Baths: Bathing is another great way to settle your spirit. Soak in a Jacuzzi, go enjoy hot spring mineral waters, or simply add some strong Dead Sea salts to your bath water at home. All of these rituals help:

- Restore moisture balance to the skin
- Provide a sense of deep relaxation
- Help relieve anxiety, stress, and tension
- Promote restfulness and sleep

Nature's Waterways: Anger is a work-out, so afterward we need to replenish our spirit, and water is always calming. Walking or sitting by the ocean, a brook, or a river, listening to nature's sounds and breathing in the negative ions are great ways to unwind and release tension. Try lying down beside a river or the pounding surf, and imagine the water running through you from head to toe, purifying your being.

Soothing Sunlight: If you feel depleted from your emotional roller coaster ride, bake away your tensions in the sun. If you're concerned about your skin, wear sunscreen, but know that most of us don't get enough sunlight. The vitamin D in sunshine has definite health benefits, and early or midday sun has been found to promote sleep and boost your mood. (Some doctors now use light therapy in conjunction with antidepressants.) You get all that, plus that wonderful feeling of just mellowing out.

WORKING THROUGH THE ANGER CYCLE:
IDENTIFYING AND INTERPRETING ANGER TRIGGERS

- List what the event or situation was and who was involved.
- Describe why this event triggered you, in detail.
- What emotions were raised by the situation?
- Is this the first time you've felt angry by this person's actions?
- What made this experience so difficult?
- What association do you currently have with this person? (Are you living together, do you interact daily, see each other occasionally, etc.)
- What association do you *wish* to have with this person?
- Do you want to maintain a connection?
- Do you wish to make amends or receive an apology?
- Are you ready to jump ship?
- Because this situation has caused you grief, have you determined what gifts you have been given as well?
- List what they are.
- List the *potential* gifts the situation can offer you.
- Is there an action you need to take to resolve this situation right now?
- Can you accept this person so that you can free yourself from the anger cycle?
- Can you forgive this person? Are you willing to do it now?

CHAPTER 9

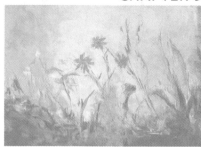

The Self-Care Equation

Nutrition and Detoxification Rituals

I've emphasized the importance of your mindset and taking time out; now, I want to talk about the Self-Care Equation, consisting of nutrition practices, detoxification rituals, and self-renewal pampering. If you haven't explored natural or alternative healing before, these practices may seem a little too involved. Or you may think they are too simple or basic to make a difference. I beg to differ! Simple works when we are in complex situations. These simple natural methods that truly restore vitality and energy back to the body lighten the load, so the immune system can work effectively.

Cleansing, fasting, and purification programs are not new trends. In today's hectic world, these detoxification rituals are needed like never before. Hippocrates, the first physician of western medicine, believed fasts were a healing mode that allowed the body to cleanse and recuperate from the impact of pollutants, toxins, and stresses of everyday life. Turns out, he was right!

Cancer and treatment are tough stuff on the body, producing toxins that need to be cleansed. Detoxification and cleansing rituals during and after cancer are like cleaning up a battlefield. Self-care after diagnosis is more important than ever, for these self-care measures can hold back and potentially reverse cancer recurrences. The ideas presented here, fit across the board if you've had surgery or not. The reason for so many suggestions is to provide the necessary support systems to clean out the toxins, so your body can win the cancer battle.

Nutrition

ORGANIC EATING

Today, when I get calls from men and women about to undergo treatment for all types of cancer, I tell them about a concept called *sacred eating*. This idea helps them lighten the load on the body by not ingesting pesticides and antibiotics found in non-organic foods, since they are already absorbing the toxic medical treatments. I let them know how important nutrition and detoxifying practices are as a pro-active step in gaining power and confidence. This gives a certain edge to the *treatable and beatable* mindset.

One of my first calls was from a woman named Agatha. She was just about to go through chemotherapy and radiation and wisely asked, "What can I do to get my body ready for these treatments? Do you have any advice?" My first response was, "You need to start drinking fresh vegetable juices daily and eating organic foods." Surprisingly, no one has ever said to me, "Oh, organic foods are so expensive" or "I don't have time to prepare fresh juices." Cancer has a way of forcing people to become more disciplined and encourages them to go that extra mile.

DIET AS A TREATMENT FOR CANCER

We all know diet is important; you can't pick up a newspaper or magazine without seeing articles on the latest diet trends. As all the research pours in, to our great frustration, the wisdom of the day keeps changing from low carbohydrates to low fat to the latest diet of the month. Many people were recently shaken when an article appeared claiming that a low-fat diet doesn't do much to prevent cancer or heart disease and another study cast doubt on the value of calcium supplements in preventing bone loss. So where do we look for the truth?

As Dr. Rubio stated in his foreword, we learn new things every day. Knowledge is dynamic, not static, so there will always be new information, and some of it will be conflicting. In sorting it all out, common sense should prevail as we look for the complete picture rather than relying on six o'clock soundbites or provocative headlines. For example, even though the value of low-fat diets per se is being questioned, we do know that obesity is a factor in cancer, diabetes, and heart disease. And too much fat puts on the pounds. The type of fat we eat is also of consequence, so it's foolish (though tempting!) to think that it's harmless to dive into a diet of cheesecake and French fries.

Here are some facts that haven't changed: *The foods and drinks we ingest give us energy and the tools we need for our cells to function efficiently and harmoniously, but the wrong foods can make us sick and cause our organs to malfunction.*

For many years, diet was ignored as a cancer-causing agent, but now we know that certain foods can be a factor in cancer and other illnesses and that our bodies are harmed by preservatives, antibiotics, and pesticides. Also, because many of us eat or chew our food improperly, we don't absorb all the nutrients we need. Our bodies contain all of the enzymes necessary to break down foods and properly absorb them. But sometimes these enzymes fail to function when they encounter foods or chemicals that they are unable to break down. This results in only partial nutritional benefits or none at all.

Many doctors use complementary medicine and work with specific diets to try to arrest cancer. Some obtain excellent results, but others get poor outcomes because their patients possess diverse genetics and respond differently to various foods. An interesting recent study has found that caffeine increases—or decreases—the risk of heart disease, depending on one's DNA. One size never fits all.

MATCHING BLOOD TYPES WITH CANCER TREATMENT NUTRITION

Diets have now been developed based on blood type that won't put additional stress on the body. Cancer patients are already under tremendous stress, so their diets should create harmony, not an additional burden.

The information in the upcoming pages is a bit technical, but it's important, so bear with me. Customized diets are important in fighting cancer because the type of nutrition the body receives can slow down or even stop the growth of cancer cells. All metabolic reactions in the cells depend on the presence of certain nutrients and water. By using the technique of matching patient blood types with diet, Dr. Rubio helps stop cancer cells from growing and assists the transformation of them back into normal cells.

Because we are omnivores (we consume both animal and vegetable substances), we need to eat a variety of foods that contain proteins, carbohydrates, and lipids to keep our bodies functioning well. A dietary regimen for cancer patients should take into account the patient's genetic constitution and should avoid upsetting the hemo-dynamics of the blood, which can cause rapid changes in the hemoglobin. Cells need nutrients, water, and oxygen to function, and the research shows that matching diet to blood types provides patients with the specifics they require.

Not everyone can tolerate a vegetarian diet because some of us need animal proteins to produce hemoglobin. Dr. Rubio found in his research that patients with O-positive or O-negative blood types require animal protein to form hemoglobin and to facilitate cellular functioning. The best sources of protein are fish low in mercury and hormone/chemical-free chicken or turkey. Patients with O-type blood also need to consume liver, which provides selenium. Liver, along with other antioxidants, produces a negative electrical charge that enhances metabolic functioning. This will slow a tumor's growth, since tumors thrive in a positively charged metabolic environment.

Patients with type A- or B-positive and negative blood can be vegetarians without compromising their hemoglobin or experiencing bouts of anemia. Patients with these blood types usually have enough selenium (an antioxidant) in their systems and do not require additional animal protein in their diets. They can also obtain the negative electrical charge useful in fighting cancer from a vegetarian diet.

THE NEED TO NOURISH EFFECTIVELY

Organic vegetables (including celery, corn, carrots, and tomatoes) can be combined with proteins, such as fish or chicken. Remember the strategy of food combining? It does make digestion and absorption easier for the body, and that is our goal while battling cancer. Food combining, simply stated, is eating proteins with vegetables or complex grains with vegetables. You don't want to mix proteins with starches, sugars, or simple carbohydrates like bread. It's too hard for the body to digest protein with carbohydrates at the same time. All vegetables, fruits, corn, and tomatoes contain hormone blockers, which also help to halt tumor growth. So just like the campaign to have five servings per day, you want to be sure to eat plenty of fresh whole foods with either your grains or proteins.

Cancer patients need extra nutrients, proteins, carbohydrates, lipids, minerals, vitamins, and enzymes in their diets because cancer cells monopolize all of the nutrients in their bodies. Cancer cells grow through the process of fermentation and don't need oxygen to survive. This is how they steal all the glucose and proteins from the healthy body and produce lactic acid. Because of their aggressiveness to survive, cancer cells can take all the nutrients and starve a body for months.

Cancer cells also switch the pH (acid/alkaline balance) in the patient's system and create a positively charged environment in which to flourish. Cancer cells have cycles: the pH in the body, normally alkaline, changes to acid when cancer cells need to nourish themselves and grow. The body's internal environment is changed, and the cancer's growth is aided. At the same time, the body's immune system is prevented from killing the cancer because a protective gel forms around the tumor cells, to disguise them from the immune system.

Cancer cells also create specific receptors to attract nutrients and specific carriers to grow and spread within the acid pH. They connect and attach themselves to normal cells and rob them of their nutrients. Cancer cells also switch electrical impulses within the bloodstream and are positively charged whereas red cells are negatively charged. Once the cancer cells steal all the nutrients from negatively charged, non-cancerous cells, they slough them off and attract new ones.

I think of this information as taking a holistic approach to the self-care equation of nutrition. Instead of being afraid, it's interesting to learn how cancer operates and then, with this awareness, to fight the battle of eating right by following your doctor's orders.

In the normal body, the pH cycle from 10 A.M. to 3 P.M. is usually acid, and from 3 P.M. to 10 P.M. it is alkaline. Then it switches back sometimes in-between. With this extra edge of knowing how cancer operates, Dr. Rubio's approach to cancer treatment is clear: *Cancer therapy must be given when the patient is in the acid phase. Any therapy given during this specific time will attack the tumor while it is attempting to grow.* Non-toxic medications and nourishment for the non-cancerous cells should be administered from 3 P.M. to 10 P.M. while the cancer cells are less active.

Cancer patients need to get all of their nutrients from the purist sources, free of chemicals or preservatives. The goals when using diet as a cancer therapy are to diminish the levels of carcinogenic agents that could adversely affect the DNA of healthy cells, to support cells as they heal, and to help the immune system function normally.

SUGAR, PROCESSED FOODS, AND CANCER

Cancer cells are nourished by sugars and nutrients that rotate to the right side. As a strategy to starve the tumor and feed the body, it's best to wean yourself off sweets for a while. Most sugary processed foods also contain chemicals. Let's use cake as a classic example of a chemical-laced food. A cake is made with fluoridated water, cooked in an aluminum pan, and frosted with icing made with artificial colors. Once ingested, millions of chemicals circulate through the digestive tract that will over-stimulate the enzymes attempting to break them down. In turn, the immune system will have to work harder to protect the body from these antigens. So processed sugary foods compete with the immune system, and this is something patients cannot afford.

When consuming any sweets during treatment, strictly limit them to the sugars that rotate to the left, like maple syrup and honeys. This provides nutrition and energy to the cells but not to the cancer. In South America and Mexico people derive energy from unbleached brown sugar as well.

ANTI-OXIDANTS PROTECT CELLS FROM FREE RADICALS

When we eat lipids (oils and fats) that are rancid, free radicals or positively charged molecules are created as the lipids are broken down into peptides and amino acids. Free radicals are positively charged molecules that are missing one electron. When free electrons interact with a cell's DNA, they can change its form and contribute to the development of cancer.

Free radicals oxidize or burn cells because of miselectrical charges. To counteract these free radicals, the most effective anti-oxidants are, first, vitamin C, followed by vitamins A and E. Good sources of anti-oxidants include the supplements grape-seed extract and pycnogenols. Negatively charged, anti-oxidants provide the extra electrons to counteract free radicals by neutralizing them and thus protecting the body's cells. These anti-oxidants are not a cure for cancer but help to protect the cells from further degeneration.

Research has shown that by adding only the anti-oxidant selenium to the diet, tumors can shrink from 8 cm to 4 cm. But it's a challenge for anyone to achieve a total cure with diet alone. Diet is only one aspect of individualized treatment.

PREVENTING CANCER THROUGH DIET

Some of the foods that defend against cancer include: broccoli, cauliflower, cabbage, carrots, other vegetables, fruits, tomatoes, ginger, garlic, fish, liver, chicken, flax seed oil, rice, beans, corn, and soy. All of these foods are high in the anti-oxidant selenium as well as vitamins A, C, and E.

Many people enjoy eating meat and fat, but they are among the biggest causes of toxins in the digestive system. I'm not saying that broccoli or carrots will stop cancer or that consuming a lot of fat will cause you to develop it, but diets rich in fat do cause the pancreas and liver to overproduce enzymes that break down fat proteins into amino acids. Also, meat sometimes contains chemicals, including anabolic growth hormones and antibiotics. Enzymes can't break down or transform these chemicals into amino acids, the building blocks for health.

All these suggestions are to help you stay focused on your self-care equation as you win the battle with cancer and then keep your healthy lifestyle going so you can feel great again.

There are various foods that tend to promote cancer growth and others that help defend the body. The following common foods are said to promote cancer growth: bacon, hot dogs, cow dairy products, cold cuts, luncheon meats, and charcoal cooking foods. If you happen to adore processed meats and barbecues, find some easy ways to make healthy and appetizing substitutions using soy products, chicken and fish, potato or goat's milk, maple syrup or honey, and herbal coffee. It's also wise to avoid alcohol, as all sugars and carbohydrates break down to alcohol at the cellular level.

VITAMINS AND MINERALS

Along with other orthodox therapies, we need to include vitamins A, B, and C in cancer treatment. These vitamins will not stop tumor growth, but they will help strengthen the immune system. They work at the same level as oxygen and DNA to combat tumors at the cellular level.

One thousand IU per day of vitamin D (compared to the currently recommended 400–600 IU) might reduce the occurrence of certain cancers by as much as fifty percent—including breast, ovarian, and colon cancer. As for risks regarding vitamin D, more than one thousand IU daily, especially if you get a lot of sun, can produce gastrointestinal problems and drive calcium blood levels too high. In addition to supplements, you can get 250–350 IU of vitamin D in a serving of oily fish or over 1,300 IU in a single tablespoon of cod liver oil. A good reference book for the specifics on nutrition is *Beating Cancer with Nutrition* by Patrick Quillin, Ph.D., R.D., CNS.

Minerals, including selenium, copper, iodine, and zinc are found in ground water. Like vitamins, they enhance the functioning of the immune system. Poor water quality and mineral deficiencies in our food chain cause our cells to become mineral-deficient and thus more susceptible to the DNA changes that cause cancer. Tumors themselves remove minerals from healthy cells.

We need a minimum of 107 minerals to stay healthy. Some we only need in trace amounts. Others are used in cancer therapy in mega-doses, such as selenium, copper, iodine, and zinc, along with calcium, magnesium, sodium, and potassium. These minerals support our body in facilitating metabolic reactions, cell reproduction, and hormone production vital to good health.

The best sources of minerals for our bodies are algae and plants grown in large freshwater lakes and the ocean. These support the body with negatively charged electrical impulses in the form of anti-oxidant substances. Algae sources produce immediate but not long-term effects in nutrition. It's important that we supplement the body with other sources of minerals and vitamins to enhance cell functioning and support the immune system.

A number of studies have shown the beneficial effects of mineral therapy. In twenty-five patients with liver cancer, tumor size was reduced when Dr. Rubio added copper to their diets. In cases of breast and uterine cancer, iodine aided the role of estrogen as a cancer blocker.

NINE THINGS YOU CAN DO

Unfortunately, it often takes a wake-up call like cancer to jolt us into becoming better informed about lifestyle choices that affect our overall health. But just as your diet may have harmed you, you can now turn it around and use it to help you heal. Here are some recommended dietary practices as given to patients at The American Metabolic Institute-Hospital San Martin:

1. Take extra digestive enzymes. Ingesting enzymes that include bromelain, amylase, and lipase combined with the hydrochloric acid already in the stomach, allows proteins to be broken down into amino acids in the digestive tract. Some people don't produce enough enzymes, they don't chew their food correctly, and they don't digest good proteins. As a result, they become poisoned by the proteins they ate to build and heal their bodies. Enzymes alleviate this from occurring.

2. Avoid drinking water with meals because it will interfere with enzyme activity; have some later after food has been digested.

3. Eat beans and brown rice at least three times a week; they contain the best combination of proteins to benefit the body. As I mentioned earlier, if you're O-positive or negative, you'll also need animal protein.

4. Cow's milk should be avoided since our systems don't have the proper enzymes to break down the proteins and end up producing more free radicals. Instead, substitute soy, goat, almond, potato, or rice milk. The same holds true for butter.

5. The best oils for cooking are sesame, canola, or olive oil; flaxseed oil shouldn't be heated but works well in salads. Oils are necessary because the body needs lipids for metabolic reactions in the cells.

6. Use breads baked without wheat, including rice bread, kamut, and oats to provide carbohydrates and energy to help maintain weight and provide fiber. Wheat contains gluten, which can be an allergen.

7. Reduce sodium intake. Many foods contain sodium, and sodium/ potassium balance plays an important role in metabolic reactions. In anti-cancer diets, salt can be obtained from garlic and celery.

8. Sugar and simple carbohydrates can produce inflammation that promotes tumor development. Chemicals irritate the colon's walls and may be absorbed into the bloodstream and re-deposited in fatty tissue—one of the prime causes of colon cancer. Laboratory studies found insecticides, pesticides, and chemicals go to the DNA level in

cells and can change their genetic code and promote the development of tumors. By instituting a proper diet based on blood type, we can help strengthen our DNA as it releases the attached chemicals and begins to heal itself.

9. Anti-cancer diets fine-tune fat consumption so the body doesn't overproduce hormones caused by eating excessive amounts of chemical-laden foods. An overabundance of hormones can also contribute to the development of breast cancer. While investigating the low rates of colon cancer in Finland, scientists discovered that the Finns ate diets rich in meat and fat but combined them with high-fiber foods (vegetables), which helped absorb and eliminate the chemicals from fat and protein-rich foods.

Detoxification

Evolving research suggests that the cause of many health problems, especially cancer, may be associated with prolonged exposure to various toxic substances in our foods and the environment. These substances can be from industrial chemicals or products, from the foods we eat and from our own altered metabolism and detoxification systems. The body's capacity to carry out this complex process of detoxification has to do in large measure with nutrition. This is why we discuss and implement proper nutritional concepts first. Certain foods can burden the detoxification machinery of your body whereas certain foods and nutrients can help it.

Many cultures around the world have long believed in the rituals of fasting and detoxifying to eliminate the underlying toxins that cause a variety of health problems. For centuries, different therapies have been used to cleanse or detoxify; from simple water fasts to sometimes elaborate regimes of bowel cleansing, steams, body wraps, and saunas.

Today, western society (and medicine) are embracing these techniques as vital to our bodily processes. Health food stores have been advocates of cleansing and detoxifying products to help people build their health. As I said earlier, it has never been more important than *now* to incorporate these disciplines into our everyday lives because in our industrialized world, we produce more and more potentially toxic compounds that find their way into the air we breathe, the water we drink, and the food we eat. The body must rid itself of these dangerous substances by transforming and then excreting them through the skin, lungs, kidneys, and bowels.

Unfortunately, not all of them get excreted efficiently—some are circulated back into the bloodstream, and others are stored in various body tissues such as fat tissue. Over the years, toxins can build up in fat, joints, the brain, and various other tissues. If you have this awareness, you can rid yourself of them by observing the suggestions that follow. Just as environmental toxins stay in the body tissues, so do the medications you take during cancer treatment. Please be sure to give yourself regular detoxification rituals, during and after cancer. During cancer treatment, detoxification rituals will assist you in getting more mileage out of your medications. After cancer, you want to build your body back, stronger, healthier, and toxin free.

THE ART OF FASTING

Under Dr. Rubio's medical care, if patients are healthy enough when they begin treatment, they start their program with a two- or three-day fast. If someone's condition is delicate, then the fast is only for one day. While fasting, patients are in a weakened but restful state. Fasting allows the body to correct the electrical imbalance caused by the presence of cancer. The metabolic reactions associated with fasting change the pH level of the blood from acid to alkaline and help prepare patients to absorb and assimilate their treatment therapies better.

Usually it's best to consume only fresh juices and teas while fasting and to eat fruit when hungry. This way, there will be continuous fluids in the stomach. In cancer patients, the body is in a catabolic phase with the cancer consuming all of the nutrients. As the radiation, vaccine, or chemotherapy destroy cancer, the wounded soldiers (i.e., dead cells) needs to be flushed out of the system. Once a three-day fast is completed, you can resume eating again—very slowly—first vegetable broth, then broth containing vegetables, soft foods, and then the recommended diet according to blood type. Slow is imperative here.

To maintain the benefits of the initial fast, a juice fast is recommended once a month as an ongoing cleansing process. If you can't quite discipline yourself for this monthly day-off-food, then take out three days to fast every three months. I think with fasting we have to experiment to find our own way. In my early treatment days I did the once-a-month plan and later on found I liked to do multiple day fasts to renew my energy.

While fasting, it's important to drink eight glasses of water daily, to flush chemicals out of the cells. Water should be filtered or purified through reverse osmosis to be sure it's free of chlorine and fluoride. Filters can also be used in showerheads to eliminate chlorine, which is carcinogenic. Having filtered water in your home is especially helpful to patients living in high chlorine concentrated areas.

JUICES AND TEAS

Our cells are typically full of chemicals; we ingest them day by day, throughout our lifetime. To help remove chemicals and support the body, it's beneficial to consume anti-oxidant-rich fruit and vegetable juices on an ongoing basis. Juices flush out chemicals that may be attached to the DNA and provide live enzymes to support good metabolic cell activity. It's good to have at least one glass of carrot juice or fresh vegetable juice each and every day during a cancer treatment program. Of course, organic is best, and this replaces sodas or the variety of chemical-laden flavored waters that are so trendy.

Herbal teas support absorption, digestion, and the maintenance of normal flora in the intestines. These will help to repress tumor growth. Recommended teas include: Pau D'Arco, Essaic, Ginger, and Slippery Elm (at least two cups per day). Green tea is also an antioxidant favorite, but during initial treatment, caffeine needs to be monitored. Noni Juice and Mangosteen Fruit Extracts are also supplemental antioxidant rich enhancers.

BATHING RITUALS FOR DETOXIFICATION AT HOME

Since the skin is the largest organ of elimination, another important way to detoxify the body is through bathing rituals and anything that makes you sweat. Steam rooms, saunas, and body wraps are lovely at spas and the health clubs, but here are suggestions for things you can do to get the medicinal effect, right at home.

During treatment I took daily salt baths to help cleanse the body and flush out the effects of radiation, chemotherapy, and the vaccine. Here is something you can do to reward yourself at the end of every day. Once you've been through whatever treatment you've had that day, give yourself the gift of a hot bath for at least twenty to thirty minutes. Here are a few tips on this detoxifying ritual: You want the water hot enough to break a sweat. After the twenty minutes are up, take a shower to rinse off any toxins you released in the water. Allow yourself to take just a few minutes out of the tub and sweat out additional impurities. This bathing ritual does take time, but it prepares you for total relaxation and a good night's sleep. Benefits include:

- Helps detoxify the body and wards off viruses
- Stimulates natural circulation for improved health
- Acts as a natural anti-bacterial
- Relaxes tense, aching muscles and joints
- Helps relieve chronic lower back pain
- Draws out impurities in the skin

At Dr. Rubio's hospital, bath salts are made from 2 Tbsp. ginger powder mixed in ¾ cup dead sea salts and a small teaspoon of baking soda. Quality matters in the type of sea salts or Dead Sea salts because there are high mineral content salts that really have a powerful medicinal effect. Anakiri Andean Mineral Salts are some of the best I've ever had. Many companies offer Dead Sea salts with aromatic oils to relax and heal as well. See Resources for more details on how to save money buying bulk salts and get the really good products. These nightly baths minimize side effects and help patients and caregivers alike.

ENEMAS ARE FOR LETTING GO

Enemas and colonics are ways to cleanse the organ of elimination, the colon. Getting all toxic medications out of this passageway is what enemas and colonics are all about. If you were ever someone who suffered from constipation prior to cancer, daily enemas may be one of the best pieces of advice you get as you go through your treatment. Check with your doctor.

Research here is good. To get you familiar with some well-known cleansing secrets: Coffee enemas have been around a long time. Coffee stimulates the liver to release toxins and helps clean the colon. The amounts vary, but 12–16 ounces of liquid, cooled down to room temperature and then implanted into the colon, should do the trick. Once you have the enema, you ideally want to wait 10–15 minutes before you let it go. Other supplements that Dr. Rubio uses for enemas are: shark cartilage, Maitake mushrooms, and colostrum enemas, which also help cleanse the colon and boost the immune system.

I recommend you talk with healthcare professionals or someone at a health food store to get the right products. You can also call the American Metabolic Institute-Hospital San Martin, where all these supplements are available for sale.

PROFESSIONAL DETOXIFICATION PROGRAMS

There is more demand than ever for detoxification practices and knowledge. Spas for optimal healing and cleansing are all over the country and the world. Special destination spas now offer weekly detoxification programs (more information in Resources) where you can exercise, have a vacation get away, and detoxify without any hassles at home.

Dr. Rubio's hospital is also well known with health professionals as a place to go for medically supervised detoxification programs. If you have a history of serious medical challenges, I do recommend medically supervised programs. Budgets vary place to place, but the new lease on life after a week-long detoxification program is worth every cent.

Self-Renewal Pampering
CREATING A HEALING ENVIRONMENT

During treatment months, you will be spending more time at home and in bed. Is your bedroom a healing retreat? Here is a lovely way to pamper yourself, by creating your vision of a healing home. Some subtle and not-so-subtle suggestions: Purchase a new bedspread, and paint your bedroom your favorite color (or any room where you'll be spending a lot of time). Purchase a print or painting that lifts your spirit and hang it in a place you'll see often. Bring plants into your room for more oxygen and life force: fountains are soothing, pillows are comforting, candles help to calm us too. Really look at your home and see what needs to be changed and do it. Before treatment, in our home we had a variety of neutral colors in our living room and dining area. The walls were a lovely shade of boring beige. When I got home from the hospital, I needed color! We painted the living room and dining area sage green then got more colorful accents in to warm the room; we still love it. Another gift to myself was I purchased some *healing art* from Aleta Pippin, a talented modernist artist who provided the image for this book cover. (Visit her gallery in Santa Fe New Mexico or website listed under Resources).

Don't forget to decorate yourself, too! Most of us spend our money on outdoor attire for business, casual wear, and workout gear. Nowadays, we need a supply of lounge wear too—women will relish this assignment. This is a great time to add to your wardrobe. In case you aren't exactly in the shopping mall mood, here are a few worthwhile catalogs filled with great ideas to decorate both you and your home: Soft Surroundings, Acacia, and Garnet Hill.

MASSAGE MINIMIZES TREATMENT SIDE EFFECTS

As part of keeping the lymph system moving and detoxifying your body, massage on a regular basis is no longer a luxury. Here is a proven way to minimize side effects very efficiently. Even after treatment is completed, many will take medications that prolong life. Thirty percent of the population will likely have to stop taking certain medications because of side effects. Here are some of the well-documented benefits researchers have found from massage therapy for cancer patients. The benefits of massage are:

- Reduce pain levels
- Reduce psychological distress
- Improve quality of sleep
- Reduce nausea
- Improve relaxation
- Improve quality of life
- Enhance body tone

Please remember that caregivers also need massage. The added stress levels can be very toxic to healthy family members, adversely affecting their own metabolic environment. So even though caregivers aren't fighting chemotherapy or other powerful medications in their bodies, they may have raised cortisol levels in the blood that impede proper functioning of many metabolic processes. Just like the cancer patient, they need to be pampered.

MOVEMENT IS LIKE A MASSAGE

The lymph is how the killer B and T cells of the immune system travel through the body. Movement is the *heart muscle* of the lymph system. It's similar to the circulatory system, but it doesn't have a pump, so we can't stay in bed all day and keep the lymph activated; we have to move. Weekly massages didn't relieve all of the soreness in my body from treatment, so I needed to keep special tabs on maintaining the lymph glands to keep moving.

I had been a workout advocate for years, so when my doctor told me to exercise, I didn't have to learn a new discipline. I did, however, hang up my Nikes and put on walking shoes. I found great relief and a way to check in with my body through weekly yoga, Pilates, Tai Chi, and other forms of exercise where mental relaxation is combined with body movement.

After a few months of treatment, something new occurred; my strength began to return, and I engaged in more frequent workouts. I listened to my body and would follow my instincts on which activities to pursue and to avoid. As I began to reemerge in activity, I'd advance a bit, sometimes plateau, then go forward again in strength, attitude, and progress. Some treatment months were more regressive than progressive, but I kept the end in mind. I wanted a fully-restored, well-functioning body.

NEEDING TO SHIFT YOUR ENERGY?

I want to emphasize that these detoxification practices are natural healing therapies that really make cancer treatment easier to handle. They may sound unfamiliar, taxing, and complex, but I hope they make a bit of sense. You want to cleanse and purify your body to lighten the load of the immune system.

After I was *out of the woods* with cancer, I noticed I would sometimes get tired or just a stuck energy feeling. I wouldn't be feeling *bad*, just not good. Often the answer for me to feel better was simple: fast, detoxify, and rest. If I just implemented these practices suddenly, I would be relieved, restored, and renewed. Life has a funny way of delivering to us valuable lessons. I now thank these healing practices for becoming valuable tools that I use to get renewed over and over again.

CHAPTER 10

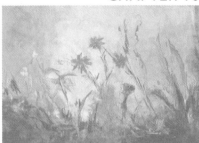

A New Approach to Life

I'm issuing a warning here: Get ready for a new view of you, once you've won the battle with cancer. This warning is for both the patient and family members. We all become educated, tested, and pushed beyond our limits while dealing with this illness. When it's finally over, how can you possibly not know more about yourself and your ability to fight for your life (or that of your loved ones). This pivotal experience rearranges your thinking. As you begin to engage in life again, there are multiple adjustments that seem to take place all at once.

At least that was the case for me, my husband, and many other survivors I know. It is one journey through cancer treatment and then another, different journey back to normal living. For advanced-stage cancer patients and families, it's been a while since you experienced ordinary life. So long in fact, that as you reacquaint yourself with normal living, it no longer feels familiar. The reason for this is—*you* have changed!

Just as your treatment took time, so does the *new you* take time to develop fully. I think that adjusting to your new approach to life can take as long as the cancer therapy, if not longer. Obviously, most people want to arm themselves against a recurrence, and to do this requires a greater sense of personal awareness—something to be emphasized over and over again.

Re-entry and Post-Traumatic Stress Disorder

I want to address Post-Traumatic Stress Disorder (PTSD), as it applies to both patients and their families. PTSD can occur following a life-threatening experience (or the witnessing of such). It is most often associated with combat veterans and disaster victims, but a grueling medical event such as cancer can have a similar impact on both the patient and loved ones. Most people recover with time, but in others the condition persists, causing nightmares and other sleep disorders, feelings of detachment, depression, substance abuse, and/or marital/familial problems.

Post-Traumatic Stress Disorder is more common among women than men and often cycles from remission to recurrence. Some patients are more vulnerable than others, depending on what your family genetics are, how many cancer recurrences you have had, other past traumas, and a variety of emotional stress factors.

For all the faith I had in Dr. Rubio and my customized treatment, never questioning my decision to just-say-no to a mastectomy, when it came to crossing the recovery finish line, I had some doubts! I soon identified these "doubts" as PTSD. I found myself compulsively checking my breasts: *yes, the lump is gone, no, it hasn't come back, wait is that a little mass or just my breast tissue I'm feeling?* Then I'd check again during my next shower. I was also over-monitoring myself by noticing my thirst levels, energy levels, and all the alarms that went off during the cancer discovery process. My mind would anxiously race: *Am I really okay? Can I really go back to a busy life and live fully again? Can I? Can I?*

In addition to psychological symptoms, PTSD can affect both the central and autonomic nervous systems, resulting in abnormal thyroid function and hormone levels that respond to stress. Although there's no definitive treatment, some people are helped by anti-depressants and others by cognitive behavioral therapy.

Breakdowns Can Create Breakthroughs

After my treatment ended successfully, I went through months where I was also prone to tears. Tears and fears I didn't express during treatment; tears of gratitude, relief, and, finally, tears of healing. I questioned myself: *Why am I so teary now that I'm cancer free?* Through journaling I arrived at this answer: *During treatment I was completely engaged in the battle for my life. Now that the battle was over, the emotions of the past years were spilling out. If I could hold on with courage and just release them, these expressions of grief...I could finally reclaim the joy of living.*

Just as soldiers instead of crying in the heat of battle show strength and tenacity, so it was with me. Once any battle is over, however, those same soldiers often need support to handle the ordeal they've experienced. We expect them to go through an adjustment phase, marked by tears and sometimes even breakdowns. And just like warriors, cancer survivors and their loved ones have endured the trials of physical torment, mental anguish, and emotional upheaval. Yet in some miraculous fashion, we have found our way back to health and life. Will we be able to accept it fully and let the past go by?

I'm not implying that all cancer survivors experience full-blown PTSD, but many do experience it at some level. I met a wonderful woman named Fran who had survived stage four lymphoma. A business acquaintance introduced us, saying, "You two should meet, as you are both survivors." The first thing I noticed after we exchanged details about our past conditions was her statement that she was "in remission." I said to her, "Having healed stage three breast cancer without any surgery, I consider myself free and clear." I pulled out my soapbox, as I elaborated. "I don't use the word remission as a way to express how I am doing today, for to me that feels like living under the shadow of cancer." Leave it to me always to express my *treatable and beatable* mindset when given the chance.

As we discussed what it was like to survive advanced stage cancer, she confided that since her "remission" she will often finds a small bump here or there, something benign, but her mind insists *this mass is cancer, the cancer is back!* She admitted that any little upset to her physical health caused her to overreact and assume the worst. This is common and part of the adjustment phase I'm referring to as we set forth our new approach to life.

I told her about my idea that PTSD often follows a cancer healing and about my own excessive breast exam phase. When I put this behavior in the context of PTSD, she got it. She understood that she could transition from this obsessive aftermath and then move on. I suggested that when asked how she was doing, she might want to affirm, "I am free and clear." We can emerge on the other side of PTSD and not live in the shadow of cancer if we allow the natural healing process to run its course.

Dare to Invite More Truth into Your Life

Each day we need to dare to invite more truth into our lives. Don't be afraid to review your past memories or hurts if they have to play out; demand to know what these situations brought to you. Be determined to receive the powerful gifts these adversities deliver. Claim them now, so you can heal and move on.

Brenda, a beautiful lady with stage four stomach cancer reminded me of this. Her oldest son had been killed in an automobile accident five years earlier, at the age of nineteen. Brenda was one of eight siblings and the strong one of the bunch. She solved everyone's problems until her son was killed. Then, slowly but surely, she shut down and knew that even though she had four children yet to raise, she wasn't the same.

Cancer came calling, and the doctors kept missing the diagnosis. When they found it at stage four, they basically said, "Go home and get things in order; you have less than a year." She arrived at Dr. Rubio's hospital and was convinced it was a miracle she found his treatment. She knew she had to fight her way back to live, and this activated her dormant strength she suppressed with the loss of her son. Watching her battle for a new approach to life inspired me.

Deepak Chopra, in his book *Quantum Healing*, references a healing phenomenon:

> Research on spontaneous cures of cancer, conducted in both the U.S. and Japan, has shown that just before the cure appears, almost every patient experiences a dramatic shift in awareness. At that moment such patients apparently jump to a new level of consciousness that prohibits the existence of cancer. This leap of consciousness seems to be the key.

It's so important to attain this new level of awareness, so we can leave the past behind and engage in a new approach to manage our lives. Once we attain this new level of awareness, we must protect it too.

Energy Lifters, Energy Drainers

In business circles, when I was returning to the business arena, people would come up to me and ask about my health. It went something like this: They would lean over and whisper in my ear, "Are you okay, dear, are you *still* okay?" Their posture and body language implied that I was in the ranks of the walking wounded. This type of greeting for me was an energy drainer.

If you want to make someone feel good after they've survived a major illness, just approach in a straightforward manner, eye to eye, extend a hand and positive greeting: *You look great; are things going well*? That's an energy lifter and far preferable to a pathetic look and—*Ohmygosh, honey, do you still have a pulse*—greeting.

A wonderful example of accepting only energy lifters into your life is a patient I met named Starr. My first question when I met her was, "Is this your given name?" And she replied, "Yes, my mother loved me so much, she named me Starr." That's an energy boost right there.

Both of Starr's parents died of cancer before they reached fifty. She was diagnosed with breast cancer five years ago and began immuno-therapy treatment. Faced with an aggressive cancer and genetics that worked against her, she chose to have surgery along with immunotherapy. During her five years of battling cancer, she has had two recurrences, but did not let up for one second on being a magnificent human being. She is a dedicated mother who home schools her two daughters, and she is a very special God-centered woman. I love this lady because she is so positive that she will *not* die of cancer.

Prior to diagnosis she had always been rather shy, but cancer gave her a new approach to life. One Sunday when she was going through treatment, Starr got up in front of the entire church congregation and announced, "If you cannot be positive and full of faith that I will heal from my current situation, please do *not* talk to me. I need to have only positive, life-affirming people around me." This was her request to her church fellowship, and it worked. She didn't need people whispering in the halls, *Is Starr going to make it?* She needed energy lifters to love and support her.

Personal Awareness Is Paramount

When I felt well enough to start back to work, I saw that I picked up where I left off: pushing myself too hard, anxious to get things moving along, and inevitably stressed. This is *not* how I thought I'd be. For all those months in treatment I was telling myself I would figure out a more "artistic approach" to business and my new life.

After a couple weeks of nearly full-time work, I was exhausted and immediately became concerned. I asked Dr. Rubio, "How can I be cancer free and still feel so weak?" His explanation was memorable: *You are like a battery that has lost its charge. All your energy went to eradicate the cancer, so now you must build back your energy reserves s-l-o-w-l-y until you are fully charged up again.* What I needed to learn was to modify my approach now that my battery was trying to get back its charge. I couldn't go full throttle now without a fallout. I'm amazed at how some of the new medicines for cancer treatment promise that patients can work during treatment or shortly after. In my humble opinion, if you have cancer, you need rest and time to tune in to your physical being.

Physical Adjustments

For some, after suffering hair loss or dealing with life after surgery, there are difficult physical adjustments to make. Quite often hair re-grows with a new texture, thick, curly, and different than before. Some might welcome this, others not. Medications can also cause numerous changes in the body. Prepare to address each change, one by one.

Are you a bit heavier? Or more fatigued? Do your joints feel stiffer after treatment? If you are heavier and stiffer, exercise will help both conditions. We need daily physical activity to flush out toxins, to sweat, and to get the heart rate up. If you're not up to something more vigor-ous, at least stretch or take a walk. Weight training helps to counter the effects of chemotherapy, as it will build muscle and strengthen your bones. Stretching is beneficial too. If it hadn't been for my yoga classes during my treatment days, I would never have made it. As the chemo-therapy made me feel old, the yoga countered the effects and helped rejuvenate me.

Minister in the Sky

After my initial ambitious attempt at returning to work, I started to weigh each commitment and assess how I felt physically and men-tally afterward. This became a form of mental gymnastics; I was nitpicking over every little ache, pain, or mental distress. I hope I don't sound psychosomatic, but there are those who ignore and those who are fixated on every little detail. I want those who are fixated to know this is a temporary condition as we transition back to normalcy.

After facilitating a spa retreat in Hawaii, I was worn out from the intense effort required to help others gain clarity and awareness (even though this is my gift and calling). This type of development work necessitates me keeping my focus on others and putting my own needs aside. After doing this for a week and being available to talk with the staff on site, I found myself about to crumble into a ball on the plane ride home. I began to question if this retreat had *taken too much out of me*, as I was still trying to recharge my battery, like Dr. Rubio's analogy.

To heighten matters, I had a two-day assignment in Palm Desert, California, as soon as I returned home.

While sitting on the plane with my brain engaged in these mental gymnastics, I noticed I was seated next to a minister and his wife. This man of the clergy was a ball of energy in his eighties. As we started to chat, I mentioned my profession. He then told me that he had recently preached four sermons on one Sunday while working in the islands. We had a lovely talk, and I was impressed with his stamina because I *know* the kind of energy it takes to do four talks in a day. I was impressed!

Since I was feeling conflicted about my health and work, I felt in need of this man's wise counsel. I told him about my cancer treatment and how worried I was about getting back into the game of life and maintaining my free and clear status. He quoted a scripture from Isaiah: "Those that wait upon the Lord shall be renewed." He also said a prayer for my complete healing before he exited the plane.

When I got home and resumed work, instead of feeling depleted from my trip, I kept repeating, "Those that wait upon the Lord shall be renewed." And when I did the two-day event in Palm Desert, I found I had the strength and stamina for the assignment.

Navigating our way to a new approach to life is tricky. Some of us err on the side of casualness and don't pay attention to symptoms. In my case I was *over*analyzing my health, energy, and durability. The minister helped me gain a new confidence and strength with which to tackle the challenges and daily activities of a full life. What an example of love and service he rendered to me that day in the sky.

Emotional Support and Awareness

Fran, the woman who survived stage four non-Hodgkin's lymphoma, had to make major changes in her relationships in order to live a healthy life after cancer. Years before being diagnosed, she had lived on the East Coast. She was preparing to move to California when her family, rather than wishing her well, said, "Why do you want to do this?" No one was supportive, least of all her very competitive sister.

As she was packing up, Fran asked this sister to please take care of her stereo until she got settled. The sister refused. Then, after her diagnosis, when she asked the same sibling for help, she was told, "If you will pay my airline ticket, I might consider coming out." The sister knew very well that Fran's cancer was serious and that the outcome was questionable. When Fran survived her treatment and was rebuilding her health and vitality back, she realized that her relationship with that competitive and unsupportive sister was not a healthy one. She ceased having regular contact with her.

I'm a Woman Who Knows What I Want

Just as Fran had to "just say no" to her sister, that is something we have to do when we are ushering ourselves back into the land of the living. One day I decided to go out to shop for a leather loveseat for our family room. I soon found the perfect one, just the right size and color. As soon as I saw that it was discounted twenty-five percent off, I approached the nearest salesperson.

After a careful inspection of the loveseat, I noticed some large black scuff marks on the back, so I requested an additional discount. The woman was very by-the-book, without much personality or humor, and gave me a curt response, "So, you're buying this piece of furniture to sell?" At that moment I knew I wasn't enjoying the purchasing process. I surprised myself by saying, "Clearly you are not *my* salesperson." As I walked away, she sarcastically scoffed, "I'm s-o-r-r-y I don't fit your sales needs." I quipped, "You didn't, and I'm a woman who knows what I want!" I purchased the loveseat from another sales associate, had a great time buying it, and it fit perfectly in our home.

As I look back, I'm not sure the first saleslady did anything "wrong" that day; she just rubbed me wrong, and being overly sensitive after cancer and all the medicines, I had (still have) my abrupt moments. But the fun part of this story was me claiming: *I'm a woman who knows what I want!* My words really hit home that day.

Social Awareness

(I MAY HAVE HAD CANCER, BUT CANCER DOESN'T HAVE ME.)

A month or so after I'd been declared cancer free, I realized that my husband's forty-fifth birthday was approaching. With all the care and support he had given me during my illness, which included everything from grocery shopping to administering injections, I knew I really wanted to make this birthday special.

A kind man had offered to fly me to Catalina in his Cessna 180 any time I wanted. Catalina Island is twenty-six miles across the sea from the Long Beach/Dana Point areas of Southern California. I hoped and prayed that it would work out as a birthday surprise for Bryan, and it did. The colorful harbor at Avalon on Catalina Island is home to a myriad of people involved in snorkeling, diving, paddle-boating, kayaking, and golf-carting. This scene made the whole day seem magical. Our new acquaintances, Howard and Denise, soon felt like lifelong friends, wishing Bryan happy birthday throughout the day. I was so grateful to be able to participate fully in this joyous event that I had dreamed of for months. I turned another corner, as I realized that having fun and participating in a social life is as important as eating well, thinking right, and keeping fit.

Laugh More—Especially at Yourself!

Finding humor in life is an art form for some people. Watch a comic, and you'll see what I mean. We may think these folks are silly or childish, but a good chuckle is often the most important thing we can give ourselves. I remember watching an interview with Bette Midler as she reminisced about an old high school friend who had increased Bette's self-esteem with her support and adoration during high school.

Here was the Divine Miss M, crying in an interview as she recalled this friend who was later killed in an auto accident. She said the two of them had laughed themselves silly all through high school and that a good laughing attack with someone is better than S-E-X. Whether you agree or not, we all know that laughter is good medicine, critical to surviving life's ups and downs.

Finding laughter again after the grimness of illness is important. It helps to laugh at temperature changes from hormone blockers or the unpredictability of one's memory after chemotherapy. Side effects are distressing, but they don't have to be unbearable.

The actor Billy Crystal brilliantly laid out his life story for laughter and healing in his book and one-man play *700 Sundays*. When Bryan and I attended the play in Los Angeles, we watched this talented and accomplished performer enthrall a star-studded audience for two hours as he revealed the troubled—as well as the good—times of his life. Each person there was able to identify as Billy took us all on a trip down memory lane, recalling his childhood and relationships.

Direct Yourself to Greatness

For all of us, now is the time to direct ourselves toward greatness. I've learned not to monitor statistics on cancer recovery, and I don't guess at how many years I have to live. I figure it's more productive to be fully alive and functioning and to make some contribution to humanity. I direct myself toward greatness and monitor my health protocol so I can achieve it.

Again, consider the wisdom of the late Christopher Reeve after his paralysis; when asked about the strain of traveling to Hollywood for his work, he remarked, "I refuse to allow a disability to determine how I live. I don't mean to be reckless, but setting a goal that seems a bit daunting actually is very helpful to recovery." I think the same is true for cancer "thrivers" as we find our way to live life anew again.

Get Ready for a New View of You!

As we realize our new approach to life, we have to let go of unrealistic expectations for ourselves and others. I know I used to feel that once I was free and clear of cancer the hard stuff would be over. Did this prove to be true? Yes and no. The *yes* is that the hard physical trials are in the past; the *no* is that as you return to the world of living fully, you may face many new challenges because the experience has changed you.

If no one is cheering you on right now...know that I am! I am cheering you on and wishing for your success. There is so much you have gained, and this is profound. You and I made it through the rain, through the pain, and survived the murky-turmoil of a brain altered by a variety of medications.

During my entire cancer healing, I was determined to make "cancer work for me." What about you? What exactly does this mean? It means we utilize the time-out from life for self-exploration and relish the opportunity to re-evaluate our relationships, projects, and our purpose in life. It was cancer that made me realize how significant relationships are and how important it is to make time for them—especially with my husband and immediate family. I also developed a new sense of personal awareness that ushered in a self-confidence I had never fully realized before.

After cancer, I was able to convey a new certainty and sense of security to my clients and audiences. I had tested my materials and message through the fires of cancer, so I knew they worked. I didn't necessarily tell my clients what I had been through, but they could feel my passion and strength. Get ready for the world to have a wonderful and powerful reaction to you. We cancer "thrivers" have a special strength, and it's just what the world needs.

CHAPTER 11

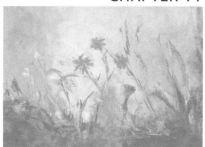

The Blessings of Cancer

H ave you ever heard the expression, *Happiness is having something to look forward to*? This idea is critical as you make your way through the dark days of cancer recovery. With a determined mindset and following the suggestions I've offered, you will have a bright new perspective for your life when the cancer ordeal is finally over. As we train ourselves to observe life carefully, we can learn to find the good that comes from adversity.

My sister-in-law was only two-thirds of the way through her treatment for breast cancer when she said, "I'm completely different now; this experience has made me realize the preciousness of life." Most patients say they are calmer after cancer when they deal with the various stresses of everyday life. That is a huge blessing in itself. We need to search for the blessings we have received as constant reminders to keep our spirits up; it doesn't matter who we are. Wherever you are in the cancer process, looking at the blessings of cancer, rather than at the downside, will help you to live a happier life.

Coping Versus Blessing

Do you tend to look at the world through rose-colored glasses or are you a worst-case scenario type? If you are the latter, this could be one area you need to change for a fulfilling cancer-free life. Destructive thoughts and words can be a deadly trap during cancer recovery. So many scare tactics swirl around this disease that we have to find a way to separate ourselves and stay clear. When it comes to diagnosis and treatment, the words used and even the way they are spoken, can propel us into a desperate state where we feel as if we must cope with our condition for the rest of our lives. Forget coping—I want blessings! Have you ever heard the saying, *What you think about comes about*?

If you really begin to focus on the blessings of cancer, you'll begin to have an attitude adjustment. This is a worthwhile cause. Here are some of the miraculous stories I've heard during my healing journey that inspired me to believe that cancer comes with many blessings to behold. I thought I'd share them with you.

Phyllis's Family Healing

Phyllis was a woman who lived a rough kind of life. She had bipolar disorder and spent many years of her life shuffling between two places; one at home raising two children as a working single parent, the other as a patient being treated in mental hospitals. While raising her children, when her condition at home would become too manic, she'd be forced to pack up her bags and become—sometimes for months— an in-patient in a mental facility.

She was always a person of faith, a spiritual woman involved in a church community. Of course, the community was aware of her condition, and as her children got older, their friends were cautioned not to get too close because of the *crazy* mother. (Some would even add to their torment by spreading rumors that the kids could be *that way* too.)

Phyllis had a strong and accomplished daughter named Courie, whom I met through a business acquaintance. We hooked up one day unexpectedly, and when I told her about my cancer ordeal, she told me about her mother Phyllis, and the blessings cancer had brought.

Phyllis was nearly seventy years old when she discovered a tumor in her breast. It had been several years since she had been institutionalized, so her *condition* stabilized. As the doctors determined that the lump in Phyllis's breast was cancerous, they immediately suggested a complete mastectomy. This was a woman who had already been through many difficult medical procedures, so Phyllis refused, saying, "This is God's way of calling me home." When she refused the surgery, the doctors institutionalized her one more time (due to her past history), saying she was *crazy to not have her breast removed!* When they finally concurred, after many weeks of observation, that she was now of sound mind, they sent her home.

Because of her mental condition, Phyllis had a social worker who visited regularly. The social worker kept a close eye monitoring both her cancer and the bi-polar disorder. With the social worker's help, when the pain got to be too much, Phyllis was admitted to a long-term care/hospice facility to die. Here is where the blessings of cancer really kicked in for Phyllis and her family.

Essentially, Phyllis claimed her power and was dying a natural death from cancer, without the side effects of treatment. At the hospice facility where she lived for a year and a half, she was described as a beacon of light to the place and its patients. The staff would go in to her room on their rounds and often, when they left her, would report that *they* felt better. She was helping the staff and ministering to patients throughout the hospital. So here is this *crazy* woman, dying of cancer and having the time of her life, *amen*!

Her daughter went to visit her and couldn't believe her mother's transformation. Here was a mother who had always been a bit of an embarrassment, now showing an amazing grace by providing friendship and giving love to all around her. Courie in the past had kept a bit of physical distance but now found herself irresistibly drawn to be together with her mom at hospice. This meant planning and packing since she was in another state and air travel was required. Courie experienced so much joy, as she shared her delightful visits, bringing her daughter, too, and enthralling the entire hospice staff.

Six visits within a year's time transformed and healed this family. Not only did Phyllis get to leave the world a respected, loved, and adored person, but also her daughter and granddaughter have the most wonderful memories to tuck away in their hearts and enjoy the rest of their lives, whenever they think of her.

People Who Need People

Does anyone not notice that the information age can have an isolating effect? A recent article on loneliness reported that people in the past claimed to have three close relationships in their lives (this is, trust-and-tell-everything friends), but newer studies have shown this number decreasing to two. For healthy working adults in our society, I'm not surprised; are you? We are usually overscheduled and overworked as we build our careers and families. We are all so self-contained by modernized society and separated by Internet access, cell phones, and instant messaging that we feel less need for personal encounters. All this *busyness* and little time for friends will create loneliness in the midst of our hectic lives. And this trend will only increase as our children, who are even more technology oriented, stay glued to their cell phones and websites such as MySpace.com. Parental interaction demands may be lessened and often unappreciated.

By contrast, think about it for a minute—who are the amazing people you have met as the result of being a cancer patient or survivor? Who are the fellow warriors you've met at the clinic, hospital or doctor's office? What stories have you shared with these people because you've been down the cancer trail together? If you have lost your gratitude and are having a difficult time with the *blessings of cancer*, I suggest you make a list of the patients you've met and the friends, old and new, who have really stood by you. Elaborate on why these people are significant. Remember the special journal I suggested you keep to document this life-changing experience? Write your list there, so you can easily review it and remind yourself of these blessings. By doing this you'll suddenly feel like the most blessed person on earth.

Roberta's New Place

Roberta's diagnosis was a catalyst that immediately changed her life. Having been raised by a minister and with years of metaphysical training, she began to use her mind constructively to visualize perfection. She made prayer a priority in her life and also transformed a guest room into a beautiful green-walled meditation room. This place was her holy-healing sanctuary where she could retreat whenever she felt the need. She included a large fountain, wind chimes, candles, plants, and tapes of bird songs. In her most terror-filled days and weeks, she slept in the room as she dealt with her fears.

Daily she spent time in prayer and meditation, affirming and talking to the tumor that was lodged behind her eyeball. Here she could also cry, rage, and release the difficult emotions of the day. This courageous minister, mother, grandmother, singer, musician, and baseball fan had her "work" cut out for her. Her treatment was a success, and she is a friend who has inspired me throughout the months and years of healing we have traveled together.

I asked her, "What was your greatest gift from cancer?" She replied, "The ease and slowing down of life. Before my diagnosis, my life was always work-oriented, rushing to get everything done. Now I take time to enjoy the little things on any given day. I now realize after cancer that I need to insert periods of recreation into my schedule." She continued, "Cancer was a difficult road to travel, because it made me face all the hurts, disappointments, and resentments I had held onto for years. However, that said, *the greatness of the rewards is commensurate with the depth of the struggle.*" As you can tell by her wise words, this is a woman who doesn't miss an opportunity to grow in spirit.

I hope Roberta's perspective will sound familiar. Both of us believe our trials in life are the fire that fashions the diamond within. Our hard knocks can bring out facets to our character that are not visible during "the good times." As part of this equation, you have to know how to pick yourself up after a hard knock and get back into the fire.

You Are Loved, More Than You Know

The actress and author Suzanne Somers was interviewed on Larry King after her non-traditional approach to breast cancer treatment. Larry poignantly asked, "There has to be some benefit in this experience; what would you say it was?" She didn't miss a beat when she said,

"Larry, I realized I was loved by more people than I knew. One morning, when it was announced I was going through treatment, a lady stuck a letter in the gated entrance of our home. I read this letter and was so touched by her heartfelt message. I knew I was loved and being prayed for by people I didn't know. What a comfort this brought to me."

I know so many people who engage in prayers for total strangers because cancer has touched their lives in some way—and what does extending a prayer cost us but a couple minutes? For those of us who have been prayed for during these tribulations, we can tell you that somehow our spirits were lifted, even though we were battling for our lives.

Earlier, I mentioned some relatives chose not to call or connect during my treatment time. Funny thing is, after all was said and done, later on relatives told me how much they were praying for me. Isn't this a true test of love?

Starr Strikes Again

One day when I was in need of some "love" to keep going on this project, I called my favorite Starr "thriver," and we had a spirited conversation. She was so elated that day and began by saying, "When I tell you this story, you will know we have so much to be grateful for!" Here is how the story goes: At my church a young man named JB was diagnosed with non-Hodgkin's lymphoma at age eighteen. He went through his initial chemotherapy treatment, and it did not work. By the time he was twenty, this once healthy and normal looking kid started to deteriorate very quickly.

His entire church community called a special prayer meeting and began to "work" on his behalf. Someone at the gathering decided to reveal his last wish, which was to marry his girlfriend. That was all they had to say, and suddenly the prayer meeting turned into a wedding planning session. The congregation became inspired and decided to make this happen. A special wedding was planned and prepared so JB could be granted one final wish, to marry his girl. This event happened within forty-eight hours!

Starr's words were so emotion filled as she recalled the impact of the event. "It was the most beautiful wedding, attended by five hundred people, all walking through this ordeal with JB. Here he was, in a wheelchair at the altar, barely able to sit up, gasping for breath with his oxygen tank by his side, unable to see his bride coming down the aisle. The best man had to whisper into his ear, 'Your bride is now walking down the aisle,' so JB would know what was taking place. Everyone wanted him to have his wedding wish, and there wasn't a dry eye in the house."

At the wedding reception, after an hour, JB looked at his bride and said, "I want to go home." Everyone at the wedding knew what was going on. The minister orchestrated it beautifully as he said, "Okay everyone, wave goodbye to JB." And they did. JB and his bride went "home" to his hospital bed. His final wish was fulfilled. JB died within the hour, with his bride by his side in her wedding gown. They clung to one another as JB left this world.

Everyone in that church community felt so connected and blessed to be a part of granting this young man his ultimate desire and sending him to his heavenly home a married man. Oh, the hearts and lives that were touched by this young man and his transition. It has been said that some people die and, in their passing, show us how to live.

Cancer Survivors Bond

My husband and I live near a country club with a park-like setting, rich with lush shades of green. Each evening we look forward to walking our dog, Lucky, and sharing the events of our day. Mornings, I do dog-walking on my own, and I always notice our fitness-minded neighbors.

There was one woman whom I saw frequently for years as we exchanged our morning greetings. She was in excellent shape, and since she would jog to my walk, I'd always encourage her. One Sunday morning, she was about to drive by, when she pulled over in her truck and announced, "You may not see me for a couple weeks—I've just been diagnosed with breast cancer." Louise knew nothing of my situation or that I was writing this book. However, she was in that very special state of shock right after diagnosis where it is not uncommon to confide in mere acquaintances and strangers.

As I listened to my neighbor, knowing she needed to get this off her chest (so to speak), I just kept observing her positive demeanor. When she told me it was stage one breast cancer, I said calmly, "You have nothing to worry about." I then mentioned I'd been through stage three breast cancer and had fully recovered.

We crossed paths several more times, and she told me she had a lumpectomy that barely changed her physical appearance. As "thrivers," we share this special bond, recalling our cancer survivors' tales. We also have the opportunity to gain insights into our own story. I knew from discussing Louise's story that if I'd been offered a lumpectomy by the surgeon that fateful day, I never would have found Dr. Rubio.

Since healing cancer without surgery is a longer process, I had to face myself in several different stages of treatment and develop the strategies in this book, to help myself and others. I chose life-enhancing cancer early on, because I didn't want to miss the blessings this adversity would deliver. I was convinced right from the start that if I'd fully experience the broad range of highs and lows, I'd learn the lessons that are unique to us all in this experience.

As cancer "thrivers," even though our stories vary here and there, we get so much when we connect. I think ultimately that is why the Breast Cancer Run and Walk for a Cure events have been so well attended. They serve an emotional bonding we survivors/"thrivers" need.

For more options to thrive, grow together and gain the blessings of cancer, visit www.treatableandbeatable.com for articles to inspire you and details about upcoming *Treatable and Beatable* Cancer Retreats throughout the country. If you want one in your own area, contact us for more details (see contact info under Resources).

As I stated earlier, I didn't write this book detailing my story so that people would no longer have surgery. I am not against procedures like mastectomy or lumpectomy or the removal of tumors or diseased organs. I wanted to address some concerns I saw in the way women and men are responding to cancer. I think as patients we need to claim our power from the moment we are diagnosed and become a part of the decision-making team.

I know one fifteen-year survivor who has experienced about every chemotherapy out there and still finds herself alive but battling with cancer after all these years. Her research on the Internet made her doctor aware of the recently approved chemotherapy pill called Revlimid for multiple myeloma, which helps build the immune system. This house-bound patient may actually be able to do her grocery shopping soon because she became part of the team in finding her solution.

I also wanted to convey to patients the importance of exploring all their options. Now that we're in the era of tailored treatment, doctors often have less time for counseling and don't want all the responsibility. There is an increasing population of people like myself who question the cut/burn/poison treatment methods and their long-term impact on health. In a poignant editorial for the *Los Angeles Times*, writer and cancer survivor Adam Baer stated, "I face many long-term effects from the 'sub-lethal' treatments I endured...10 years later I have mysterious health issues that are most likely the results of my so-called cure. And no one knows what to do." So to those who want to make surgery and/or potent chemotherapy a last resort, I hope you'll now know that you have a choice.

Since surgery is a non-reversible solution, these stories have been given to illustrate that less invasive options do currently exist. Some of you may have to leave the country, but lawsuits challenging the status quo are occurring all over the United States; research, and you will find out about them.

We are in charge of our lives; becoming part of the decision-making process helps maintain the *treatable and beatable* mindset. Instead of being told what to do like small children, we are planning our future together with our medical team. We can honor our beliefs and intuition when it comes to deciding on the treatment regimen and the medical team we want to work together with. This brings me to a an-other reason why I wrote the book: to encourage people to gain greater personal awareness and power as a result of cancer. Elizabeth Edwards (wife of Senator John Edwards) demonstrated this when her breast can-cer metastasized and she went on the campaign trail anyway!

Watch for the Shining Moments

My husband recently went in for an annual checkup, having had chest pains on and off for months. Right there in the doctor's examina-tion room the chest pains began again. The physician was concerned that it might be a heart attack and called the paramedics. When I was informed that Bryan had been rushed to the hospital, I dropped every-thing and joined him immediately.

Once I saw him all hooked up with monitors and wires, I realized that I was now going to experience what it's like for the caregiver in a critical situation. Here was my husband, used to taking care of me, and now he was the one enduring pain and experiencing the mental impact of feeling helpless. He immediately said, "I hope I was nice enough to you during your treatment—this is horrible." Of course, he had been, but now he was seeing firsthand the obstacle course I had lived through.

After hours of waiting to be admitted, I left him at the hospital to go get food and walk the dog. Just leaving the hospital, there was this heavy weight of concern and worry with my every step. Suddenly, I saw how enormous his task as a caregiver had been. Even if you are healthy, as a caregiver, you feel sick at heart when your loved ones are ill.

When I returned to the hospital, Bryan was still in the emergency area, and he said softly, "It has been hectic here. A twenty-five-year-old girl has just been admitted on the other side of the curtain." He contin-ued in a whisper, "She attempted suicide." He told me it had been an eventful couple hours, and he could overhear all the attempts to revive her.

As the nurses were attending to the now-conscious girl, one of them scolded her when she asked to see the social worker. She said, "You don't feel good because of the pills *you* took. A counselor is coming to see you, but she's busy right now!" There was little sympathy, and her tone suggested, "*You* got yourself into this mess."

Being so close to this situation and hearing every word, I said to my husband, "I either have to go over and talk to her or I have to leave." He didn't want me to get involved in a potentially sticky situation, so he suggested I get some dinner and bring something back to him. I started to leave, but as I walked by the girl's bed, I stopped and asked, "Can I pray for you?" She looked up at me with these gorgeous turquoise eyes and said, "Yes."

She told me her name was Jenny. I couldn't help staring into her eyes, and I just came out with, "Jenny, you have a lot of life left in you; you're a very pretty girl." Her eyes encouraged me, so I continued, "But what you have yet to learn is that sometimes when things seem desperate and unbearable, that's when a shining moment or miracle is just around the corner. You have to learn to live through those dark and desperate days to see what solution or answer life is going to bring your way." She smiled slightly as I went on. "In my opinion, the spectacular part of life is comprised of these shining moments. The rest is like a circus, and you just have to take it in or let it pass by."

She began to tell me of her desperation, and to my amazement, the nurse who had been scolding her returned with an IV and didn't confront either of us. So I continued, "Please, relax yourself now. Your body has been through quite an ordeal, and the best thing you can do at this moment is to just relax." I thought the IV probably contained a sedative, so it seemed as if her shining solution might be starting to emerge.

What happened that day was a *blessing of cancer* for me. I was able to go to her because I knew the suffering firsthand from my dark and difficult times. I knew her desperation. This qualified me to offer a hand to someone who wasn't a cancer patient, but just another human being in a desperate situation. As I reflect back, had I not followed my urge to reach out to her that day, I would have missed out. I was still distressed by my husband's situation, but every time I thought of Jenny,

I knew I had a shining moment tucked under my sleeve to carry me through.

Greater Compassion

After all is said and done, one of the blessings of cancer is the greater compassion we can offer patients and families who are suffering. I actually think this is part of the assignment if we are fortunate enough to fight our way back from life-threatening illness—that we learn to pass along our compassion and hope.

Consider again the women who volunteer and coordinate these three-day breast cancer events across the country, raising money to find a cure. These people, mostly survivors and loved ones, have found a new meaning to life and want to give others help. Sometimes, as cancer "thrivers," we have the upper hand when it comes to meeting the emotional needs of other patients and those who are suffering. We seem to expect doctors and nurses to *do it all*, yet they are the ones who have to coordinate all the details of our treatment and save our lives. That is a tall order and an immense task right there.

I think Dr. Rubio is unique, for although he is just as rushed as any other doctor, whenever he gave me an update or advice on my next course of treatment, he conveyed an enormous energy of confidence combined with a sense of calmness. There were times when I was low or even desperate, and during a routine visit he would somehow transform my fear into hope. After his visit, I would feel like *I'm going to beat this cancer*; now that is what I call *Good Medicine!*

True Self-Authority and Efficacy

Self-efficacy is a person's belief in his or her capacity to achieve something and the power to produce an intended result. To really believe in one's self is the greatest wealth on earth. When I believe in myself, I can have it all, because I believe I can. Believe in your cancer healing. Have a vision of your life after cancer as glorious and fulfilling.

When you believe your life has purpose (which it does even if you don't think so), then there is some purpose in you having cancer, even if it is not readily apparent. Be inspired to find greater self-awareness as you go on making your life worth living; find a purpose. Cancer is an opportunity for a better life. Please don't let this opportunity to learn more about your strengths, fighting spirit, resilience, and adaptability slip away.

I decided to use my cancer experience to set a new course for my life early on. I did this by claiming my power, exploring options that fit for me, and seeking to find a greater meaning in my life. We have to listen to our hearts, minds, and bodies when it comes to taking medicines or submitting to harsh treatment protocols. As Dr. Rubio states in the foreword, a patient is the captain of his ship, and your body is the vessel he speaks of. Before I met him, I was already acting like the captain of my ship, searching for someone with his talent and forward-thinking treatment methods. I hope you will benefit from the emotional and mental aspects of my story as I "held the course" and healed my life. I ask you all to notice the good you have received from this experience—this is the treatable and beatable mindset—and expect many more magical blessings of cancer!

Sitting on the Edge of a Dream

Sitting on the edge of a dream:

Is this what all the hard work means?

One day it comes, and you succumb;

You're sitting on the edge of a dream.

Sitting on the edge of a smile;

Sometimes it takes awhile.

Depends upon the situation or trial;

But there you are one day,

Sitting on the edge of a smile.

Sitting on the edge of your life:

Did it make sense?

Or was it filled with strife?

You search for meaning, dreams, and smiles.

Sometimes it takes awhile.

—*Carolyn Gross, August 2006*

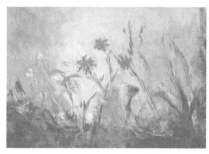

Epilogue:
A Special Message for Caregivers, Families, and Friends

Cancer's effects are far-reaching, and eventually it touches us all. Every one of us knows a parent, grandparent, sibling, friend, or family member who is now battling cancer or has been a patient in the past. Here are some suggestions for friends and families. If you can interact well with your cancer-challenged loved ones, your support and ability to roll with the punches will ultimately make you a stronger and wiser person.

Let the Patient Choose

I've talked about the power of choice in Chapter One. Most patients, when first diagnosed, don't realize they have options, although that is quickly changing. The patient and their doctor of choice should decide the course of treatment. If you, as a friend or spouse interfere here, you could have some serious regrets down the road. If you have a loved one who decides not to participate in all or parts of the traditional treatment protocol, please don't pressure him or her into surgery or chemotherapy or whatever procedure that person might wish to avoid. Don't use the kids as an excuse or *What will happen to me?* if they don't choose the course you think is best. Each life is precious, and each patient's choice must be honored. If you're having trouble with this, reverse the scenario in your mind; if you were the patient, how would you feel?

I'll be forever grateful that my husband didn't oppose me when I elected to work with Dr. Rubio, instead of opting for traditional mastectomy surgery. He hesitated at first, but once he'd met with Dr. Rubio, he was more comfortable with my decision. Bryan remembered all too well his own mother's experience when she was diagnosed with breast cancer. She had a mastectomy, as advised by her doctor, but her cancer later spread to her brain, and she was dead at fifty-two. He was familiar with her treatment and understood that there are no guarantees. His knowledge and background enabled him to be supportive and involved in my post-treatment home care program.

Since I don't recommend coercing or cajoling, here are some things you can do to help: You can do research, locate recommended doctors, make phone calls, and help set up a support network. Once you're up to speed on the latest treatments, you can share your knowledge with the patient, showing love, concern, and compassion. But always leave the final choice to him or her.

Be a Good Visitor Rather Than the Guest from Hell

Visiting a new patient is not always an easy task. Cancer complicates a person's life in a number of ways and dramatically increases the unknown factor. It's initially unknown whether the treatment is working. It's unknown whether the person will pull through or not. There are so many variables—all out of our control. What *is* known is your affection for this person, and the point of the visit is to share your fondness and good wishes. Take it from me: The last thing any cancer patient needs to hear is how you lost some other friend to the disease.

So how do you prepare for a visit when at a personal level you are really frightened for your friend, yet don't want your fears to show? Try to make your visits selfless. When you see him or her, be open to serving the patient's needs rather than your own. You may not know in advance what those needs are, but if you're intent on brightening that person's day, you'll be surprised what can happen.

I recently visited my dear friend Judith, who has battled cancer for over fifteen years. Even after chemotherapy, stem cell therapies, and experimental drugs, her cancer returned. When she discovered that the new medicines weren't working, I had to put my own fears aside and concentrate on her needs. Prior to the visit I was nervous; *was she close to being on her death bed?* When Judith answered the door, the answer was clearly *no*. However, as we had tea and talked that day, I suspected that, having lived in the shadow of death for over two years, she was now wondering just how horrific this next episode might be.

In the spirit of service, I found words that sprang from my heart: "Judith, this experience could be a new beginning or an ending. Let's just assume that your suffering is in the past. To experience incomprehensible deterioration or demoralization is an illusion. You've already done that work. Let's just give this need for healing to the multitude of angels ministering to you now, so you can rest peacefully."

Judith is a minister, so these words were apparently just what she needed; her face lit up when I'd finished speaking. For all the anxiety I experienced prior to the visit, when I left I was walking on air. This is an example of what is possible and the immensity of the experience for both of you, when you visit with love and selflessness in your heart.

When to Be Honest—And When to Bite Your Tongue

There's a certain pressure to put on a good show when visiting someone who is ill. We need to be strong, but if we put on too much of a facade, the patient will end up feeling the disconnection. The best way to help a loved one heal is to be honest, caring, and most of all, sensitive. Laughter is wonderful, too!

One caveat: There are times when too much honesty can do harm. If, for example, you should have an emotional meltdown in front of a sick friend, it's important to learn the effect of your behavior. If you find that you've upset the patient, then in the future it's critical that you process your true feelings elsewhere and prepare ahead of your visit with selflessness in mind. However, if it's clear that your strong emotions made her feel loved and cared for, then just let your feelings flow.

When visiting, it's important to focus on the positive: *Your attitude is so good; you have a sparkle in your eyes!* These spoken encouragements are helpful and welcomed. Just as this book suggests that patients pursue a *treatable and beatable* approach, so should family and friends. Offering condolences in a pathetic tone is *not* a good approach. A dramatic tone implies the worst and is likely to fuel already existing fears. When visiting patients in their homes or the hospital, look for the positive and reinforce it with your comments.

That said, it's important to be sensitive to the patient and to respond accordingly. Some cancer patients have reported feeling burdened and resentful when loved ones are relentlessly cheerful. Occasionally, it's even implied that if a patient isn't doing well, it's because he or she isn't trying hard enough—a shameful version of blaming the victim. Although a positive attitude is generally desirable, one should never force a patient into faking false emotions.

Some of us are more at ease than others with our own mortality. If your loved one wants to discuss end-of-life issues and you feel threatened by such discussions, it's not a character flaw—you're just not the person to help him or her in this particular way. Perhaps you can recommend a professional or another friend who can provide the support they need at this time.

Finally—always use common sense. One of my neighbors visited me after I had returned home from Dr. Rubio's hospital. She walked in the door and placed her hands on my face and chirped, "Oh my goodness, your face is so round and chubby!" In my weakened state, and after years of struggling to keep a stylish figure, you can imagine how that went over. To me it sounded like, *Honey, you've got cancer* and *you're fat!* So before you rush in and state the obvious, make sure your tongue has a working relationship with your brain.

The Best Gift of All

It's good to remember that most cancer patients are formerly active people who are now more or less under house arrest. What would brighten *your* day if you had to switch places? Patients going through treatment generally need help with shopping, meals, babysitting, doctor visits, and creative recreation.

There are many ways we can show our love, but practically speaking, the greatest gift of all may be *organization*. I recently heard about a young mother who was devastated when she learned that she needed immediate surgery to remove a rapidly growing tumor. She sent emails to friends and relatives stating that she would need full-time help during her recovery. The response was overwhelming—within hours she was flooded with expressions of love and offers of food and assistance. But, as heartwarming as this might sound, Sarah could easily have ended up with twenty hot meals sitting around incubating E-coli and a dozen babysitters clamoring in her living room. Fortunately, one of her forward-thinking friends sent emails to everyone on the team, allowing these generous gifts of food and time to arrive in a timely and truly helpful fashion.

Many of us have a circle of relatives and friends from various areas of our life, but these folks rarely all know one another. If one or two capable people can put them in touch (thank God for email!), it's not hard to organize an effective team, with many people providing support so that no one person becomes overburdened.

The Challenges of Care Giving

I talked about Kerri and her husband earlier in the book. During the ups and downs of her husband's three-year battle, she told me this: She became a better person, she learned to be more patient with difficult situations, and when she listened to people complain about mundane problems, she'd smile and think to herself, *You have no idea what hard times are!*

As mentioned above, sometimes you have to table the upbeat approach and just roll with the situation. It's important not to push the patient when he or she is clearly not ready or in the mood. Kerri explained that after Raul had endured three chemotherapy treatments, his mood would change when he arrived at the clinic. This normally high-spirited, gregarious guy became glum and withdrawn. "Once the treatment was over," she said, "he was fine, but often he'd become short-tempered and not himself while the procedure was taking place." As a caregiver, this is not the time to interfere. This is where the added patience that Kerri developed can be so valuable.

Ask for the Help You Need

Not all of us, however, are blessed with endless patience, and care giving can be a long, arduous, and complex task. In a world where we're all living longer, it's not unusual for someone to be caring for a sick spouse or sibling as well as an elderly parent. Again, this is where shared efforts can make a tremendous difference. When one person bears all the responsibility, the price is grim; studies show that primary caregivers have shorter life spans, and some even die before the people they're caring for.

The solution is never simple, but with ingenuity and persistence, the impossible can become manageable. Soliciting the help of family, friends, neighbors, and professional caregivers, and asking them to each contribute a small gift of time can do much toward relieving the person in charge.

I'd like to share some thoughts about hospices: Many people cringe at the idea, thinking that the very mention of the "H-word" means giving up and, even worse, sealing a loved one's fate. But that is simply not the case. It's not at all unusual for patients to be placed in hospice care and then recover enough to say *See you later!*—to the delight of everyone. In the meantime, respite care and support to the family have been provided. One friend I know even called a hospice when she was in desperate search of a rehab facility for her father. She told them upfront that hospice services were not required at that time, yet she was given immediate and invaluable information about local resources.

So don't rule out any*one* or any service. There is a lot of help out there available at little or no cost. The most important thing is to *ask* for the help you need.

Whatever One's Beliefs, You Can Offer a Prayer

In today's diverse world, most of us interact with people of all faiths, and we learn to respect each other's beliefs and customs. The common threads most religions and spiritual traditions honor are prayer and meditation. Even those who consider themselves atheists are unlikely to be offended by offered prayers, as this is a universal symbol of love and support.

If prayer is one of the ways you wish to help a loved one, don't take the assignment lightly. Some people think that careening through traffic while mumbling, "God bless my friend," is a good enough way to pray. I beg to differ; that's what I call *the multi-tasker's prayer.* I think when it comes to this type of appeal, we need to send our *focused* love and power to those in need.

If you happen to be accompanying your friend to a doctor's visit or while waiting for test results, you might want to concentrate silently on some affirmative thoughts: *This is all working out for the highest good. The hand of God will be present in the physician's treatment today and always.* In the silence of your being, you can pray as you wait.

If you feel you aren't up to the task of praying on your own, consider giving the patient's name to a prayer circle. One of my favorites is Unity. They have a prayer tower open twenty-four hours a day, seven days a week. This is not a recorded message, but a live person, awaiting your prayer request 24/7. You can call anytime, and someone will pray with you immediately and then put your request into their prayer tower for thirty days. This is a wondrous service. I always call them with the major challenges I can't handle on my own. Their number is (816) 969-2000 or, toll free, (800) 669-7729. If you can afford it, you might want to send them a donation, before, during, or after a prayer request.

If your medical bills are such that you need to feel you can manage and attract prosperity in your life, here is another great phone number: Catherine Ponders Dial-a-Thought at (760) 346-3964. Her pre-recorded message will give you a prosperity lift. She wrote the book *Open Your Mind to Prosperity*, and it's a classic!

Just as patients need a treatable and beatable mindset, caregivers have to excel in flexibility, tolerance, and offering a stable environment for patients to recover in. If that stability comes from the consistent support of family and friends, that is the best care giving around.

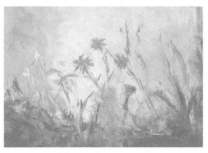

Afterword:
Customized Cancer
Vaccines Heal the
Body from Within
by Geronimo Rubio, M.D.

C ancer vaccines are one of the hottest areas of research in the United States, with many promising studies showing positive results in treating disease conditions. A recent vaccine for cervical cancer is the first one to emerge in the U.S. market. All over the world, doctors and biologist are beginning to study and recognize immunotherapy as a viable treatment option. At American Metabolic Institute-Hospital San Martin, we have included this treatment protocol for over twenty years, and it forms the heart of our cancer treatment program.

Through developing a series of remarkable vaccines from components of the patient's own body and cancer cells, we have discovered that vaccines can impart information to the natural defenses to stop and destroy cancerous tumors effectively. This is how Carolyn Gross and thousands of other patients have recovered. Immunotherapy enhances the body's unique ability to heal itself from within. Some patients use immunotherapy as an adjunct to surgery they have in the United States, to enhance the body's ability to maintain a cancer-free environment.

When properly awakened, a patient's immune system already has all the tools necessary to detect, attack, and destroy cancer. The only way to stop cancer completely is through enhancing the immune system's functioning. To achieve this goal, the immunotherapy protocols developed have been proven effective time and time again, especially when used in conjunction with low doses of chemotherapy and radiation.

Customized Treatments Boost Immune Functions

Cancer requires doctors to work individually with each patient. Each person has an individual map for healing and recovery, and we need to discover this map or code to make therapy programs work, physically, mentally, and emotionally for each patient. My aim has always been to work out an individual program of patient care and to recognize the constant metabolic changes taking place internally. Our bodies are constantly in transition, so the best treatment methods involve vital therapies, such as these individualized vaccines created from the patient's own proteins.

Our protocol begins by simultaneously administering the vaccines along with low doses of chemotherapy and radiation to wipe out the tumor so it has less of a chance to change form and return. We peel away the protective protein coat and expose the tumor, which allows the immune system to attack it intelligently. There's a much better success rate than would be expected using only traditional treatments.

Chemotherapy and radiation do, however, offer substantial benefits to the cancer patient. They allow an enhanced immune system to work against fewer cancer cells and increase its chances of destroying the tumor. With cancer, the immune system may be overwhelmed, with one fighter cell waging war against perhaps twenty-five cancer cells. The immune system has little chance of winning; sooner or later the cancer will kill the host.

Through immune-enhancing therapies, we increase the number of immune system cells from five billion to, say, perhaps seven billion cells. At the same time, the low doses of chemotherapy and radiation work to reduce the number of cancer cells from twenty-five billion to ten billion. By making the playing field more even, we know this gives the patient a better chance for success.

The Immune System at a Glance

Our immune system is the defense mechanism that protects us against the negative influences of antigens, proteins, bacteria, chemicals, and cancerous cells that can cause us to become sick or develop diseases. It is composed of various types of white blood cells called lymphocytes, whose numbers increase in response to infection and disease, including cancer.

There are two primary types of immunity in the body: humoral, composed of B-cells, which produce antibodies that attack foreign cells, and the cellular, composed of T-cells, which react to and attack specific foreign substances or viruses. Both components are formed principally in the bone marrow, with the T-cells maturing in the thymus.

Killer T-cells attach themselves to specific foreign cells and secrete substances to destroy them. They make up about twenty-five percent of all T-cells in the body. Helper T-cells secrete interleukins, interferon, and other immune proteins to stimulate B-cells and killer T-cells to attack foreign invaders. About sixty-five percent of all T-cells are Helper T-cells.

Suppressor T-cells turn off excessive reactions by the immune system and suppress activity of the antibodies.

Still another type of white blood cells is the Natural Killer (NK) cell. Natural Killer cells are neither B nor T-cells, but are equipped with an arsenal of up to one hundred different poisons to recognize and kill foreign invaders quickly. All of these components of the immune system work to galvanize the inner systems of the body and quickly scour it of foreign cells and antigens.

Immunotherapy Educates the Immune System

The immune system is empowered to stop any illness in the body. However, with cancer patients there's a breakdown because the immune system fails to recognize the cancer as an abnormal growth. The body's natural defense mechanisms are unable to recognize a cancerous tumor because it hides behind a specific camouflage, a protein coating that acts as a blocking factor. The immune system does not recognize the protein as foreign, sensing instead that it is a normal protein and, thus, leaves the cancer alone.

An important first step before we use any kind of immunotherapy is to destroy the camouflage and expose the cancer cells. We utilize techniques to break the protective protein coating by imploding it—making small holes in it. The best method utilizes specific protolytic enzymes and amino acids with specific carriers. This way, we expose targets on the tumors and create pathways for the immune system to attack.

The next step is to administer vaccines, to educate and direct the immune system to attack and destroy the tumor. An additional benefit of the vaccine is that the educated T-cells will send messages to the patient's bone marrow and direct it to produce copies of the same type of T-cells to attack the cancer.

When treating patients, we use five different types of vaccines to train the immune system to attack the cancer: the Passive Vaccine, Active Vaccine, Non-specific Vaccine, Specific Vaccine, and Dendritic Vaccine. American Metabolic Institute-Hospital San Martin is one of the few cancer treatment centers in the world where they are *all* available.

Passive Vaccine

The Passive Vaccine works to eradicate any type of cancer in the body. Within three to five weeks after the vaccine is administered, there is often a reduction in the tumor's size, as well as in the intensity of any accompanying pain. The reason for my vaccine research these last twenty years is because chemotherapy and radiation may shrink and stop the tumor for a while but will not destroy it completely.

This Passive Vaccine works to destroy cancer totally. Because it is created from proteins extracted from the patient's own body, it doesn't cause as many devastating side effects as do traditional chemotherapy and radiation. After the vaccine is injected, patients might experience a fever, muscle aches, and headaches for forty-eight to seventy-two hours.

These symptoms are not side effects; they are symptoms that occur because a lot of activity is taking place internally. (Medically speaking, we call these symptoms *pirrogen endogenous*.)

The Passive Vaccine was developed to facilitate a process we call RNA transference of the lymphocytes. In the RNA transference, one white blood cell transmits information to other white blood cells to attack the cancer. Essentially, we are multiplying the army of educated cells that will attack and destroy the tumor.

The process for creating RNA transference of the lymphocytes takes twenty-one days in the laboratory. These white cells now have the memory and the ability to recognize the tumor and attack it. Taking the educated white blood cells from a culture created, we inject them back into the patient's bloodstream. By this time, specific washing factors and protocols have already been employed to penetrate the cancer's protective protein coat. The educated white blood cells, which have memorized the cancer's protein make-up, are attracted to the exposed tumor to attack and destroy it, as well as any similar metastasized cancer cells.

The effects of the Passive Vaccine last up to three months. After three months, the RNA transference of the white blood cells starts to decline, and the vaccine has to be repeated. As the number of T-cells diminish, more cancer cells escape the immune system, change their protein composition, and escape from the beneficial effects of the vaccine.

It is at that time we have to repeat the process because the cancer becomes resistant and transforms itself while fighting for survival. To survive, the cancer will change its protein coating and its cells will be altered. To continue with the healing process, we need to keep the immune system informed and updated.

During the past twenty years of using the Passive Vaccine, combined with low doses of radiation and chemotherapy, we've witnessed remarkable results, and patients respond one hundred percent better with the vaccines than through the use of traditional treatments alone.

It is my estimation after working with Passive Vaccines and Dendritic Vaccines that they are the most effective of all our cancer therapies.

Non-Specific Vaccine

Since the advent of medicine, doctors have attempted to work intelligently to stop illness by using tools that enhance the body's innate healing abilities. Through this research, they have found that using different compounds can awaken or stimulate the immune system.

In the use of Non-specific Vaccines, as the name implies, we stimulate the immune system in a general way to increase the number of white cells and stimulate their motivation to attack a specific target. We create Non-specific Vaccines by combining different types of lipids from bacteria. These lipids are strong immune system boosters.

To administer the vaccine, we inject different types of bacteria in a non-active state under the skin. We've seen these lipids grow in a manner similar to the way cancer grows. When we apply the deactivated bacteria, the capsule of lipids grows and then competes with the tumor, both for space and nourishment, and helps starve the cancer cells. The lipids around these bacteria also stimulate the immune system to increase the production of white blood cells. The strengthened immune system can then take advantage of the tumor in its weakened state and begin working to eradicate it.

This sets the stage for the RNA transference process three weeks later with the Passive Vaccine. The process is similar to tuning the engine of a racing car before the race. Vaccines created with lipids from deactivated BCG/tetanus can also be used like an insurance policy to prevent the development of cancer. In countries such as Mexico and South America where children are vaccinated with the BCG vaccine when they are born, the incidence of cancer is much lower. It seems the BCG vaccine protects the body from developing tumors later in life. BCG vaccines have been in existence since the 1840s when they were developed against tuberculosis, but now have fallen out of use in the United States.

Our research in clinical practice has shown that application of BCG as an immunotherapy is effective for melanomas and against *all* cancer when used in conjunction with low doses of chemotherapy (Vincristin) and specific hormone blockers. High doses of chemotherapy are unnecessary; through these therapies alone we have been successful in putting the bone marrow into complete remission.

Again, in conjunction with the Non-Specific Vaccines, we incorporate a strong detoxification program and use the Rife Frequency Generator to maintain control over the tumor. Using the Non-Specific Vaccines with breast cancer, combined with hormone blockers, we've witnessed a rapid reduction in tumor size, as was the case for Carolyn.

Non-Specific Vaccines are applied at the hospital during the first week of therapy, following completion of the first segment of the diet and nutrition program. They are an immune system booster that sets the stage to support the Passive Vaccine in the weeks that follow.

Active Vaccine

Active Vaccines are an amazing technique to activate and direct the immune system against tumors. For a long time, doctors have worked with these types of vaccines and witnessed remarkable responses. A specialty at our institute, we make this vaccine *specifically customized* for each patient.

To formulate the Active Vaccine, we obtain a piece of the tumor from the patient through surgery or a needle biopsy. When we cannot obtain cancer cells, we use antigens from the blood or urine to make the vaccine. We remove the protein coat from the extracted tumor cells and apply a low dose of radiation to slow them down and kill them. At the same time, we are careful not to destroy the DNA or genes of the cancer. We then add specific lipids and polypeptides to the dead cancer cells and inject this combined substance back into the patient under the skin and intramuscularly.

This preparation produces an immediate reaction in the patient's body as T-cells and hordes of white blood cells rush to the inoculation site and begin to attack and destroy the foreign protein, lipids, and polypeptides. This activation against these foreign-looking proteins and lipids stimulates the immune system to recognize the tumor as a foreign body and to begin a program to attack and destroy it.

The Active Vaccine also stimulates the bone marrow to produce and send even more T-cells to attack the foreign proteins and lipids. While attacking the strange proteins, the activated immune system will also attack the proteins of the cancer and will search throughout the body for the same strange proteins as metastasized cancer cells in the liver, brain, or lymph glands.

Typically, we use Active Vaccines during the second week of therapy. It is most effective with solid tumors, adenocarcinomas, melanomas, sarcomas, and cancers of the breast, stomach, lungs, and colon. It prevents tumor growth by blocking the formation of new blood vessels to nourish the tumor.

As with the other immune system boosters, the Active Vaccine supports the strongest vaccine, which follows as the end of the third week: the Passive Vaccine. Combining these therapies, we see a dramatic change in tumors and an accompanying reduction in pain. The immune system becomes stronger, more alert, and more functional, providing an opportunity for the cancer to be destroyed.

The Active Vaccine works synergistically with all the other therapies, including chemotherapy, radiation, herbs, and natural methods and has been successful working specifically with melanomas. We've seen patients with melanomas that have spread to the bones, liver, blood, and brain respond to the Active, Passive, and Non-Specific vaccines combined with interferon. The pain diminishes, and the tumors stop growing. With adenocarcinomas, lymphosarcomas, and leimasarcomas, we also see dramatic changes and the tumor arrested.

Specific Vaccine

For the past sixty years, doctors, biologists, and chemists have experimented with different types of bacteria to try to awaken the immune response. The Specific Vaccine works by introducing live bacteria within the body to compromise the tumor by creating a competitive environment for nourishment and territory. To make the vaccine, we can use active staphylococci, pneumoccoci, or clostridium tetanus. We need to recall that our bodies already function as a culture for many kinds of funguses and viruses, and in some cases we can use this environment to our advantage.

Specific Vaccines need to be applied carefully in difficult situations and in specific cases. They are especially effective when it is difficult to reverse a large tumor or when edema does not respond to other therapies. The Specific Vaccines can be used daily or weekly in a safe way to stimulate the immune system to create more white blood cells and prepare the patient's body for the next series of vaccines.

Dendritic Vaccine

Dendritic cells have the assignment of killing all the antigens on the cancer cell surfaces. It has great impact by sending messages to the immune system to destroy tumors, and this vaccine works well with all types. The dendritic cells are heavy hitters, displaying those antigens to the killer T-cells through an incubation process.

This vaccine is customized by again extracting some of the patient's dendritic cells with immune cell stimulants to reproduce large amounts of dendritic cells in the lab. These cells are then exposed to antigens from the patient's cancer cells. This combination of dendritic cells and antigens is injected into the patient, and the dendritic cells work to program the T-cells. The process is similar to that of the Passive Vaccine.

The Dendritic Vaccine is a more recent discovery using the genetic code of proteins produced in cells to aid the immune system. Bits of DNA from the patient's cells are injected into the patient, which instructs the other cells to produce certain antigens continuously. This DNA vaccine increases production of antigens, which forces the immune system to respond by producing more T-cells.

If The Tumor Is Not Removed, Where Does It Go?

While the vaccines are working, the white blood cells are attacking the tumor, and the tumor is starting to die. You may ask, what happens when the tumor dies? Where does it go? The tumor liquefies or breaks down into small pieces. The protein fragments enter the bloodstream and are processed through the lymph system.

The lymphatic system begins to overload with the waste as T-cells encapsulate pieces of the tumor; they are processed through the lymph system and re-deposited in the bloodstream. The dead tumor cells, protein poisoning, and other wastes from the process are then eliminated through the kidneys, liver, colon, and skin.

Patients and doctors need to be aware that when we destroy tumors, we are creating protein poisons and free radicals. It's important to detoxify these organs of elimination both before and after treatment to allow them to function optimally to drain wastes from the body.

The immune system is the key that unlocks the door to a successful recovery from cancer. Based on my research, the entire focus of cancer treatment programs should be to support and enhance immune functioning through creating an ideal cancer-fighting environment within the body. As a doctor, I've witnessed amazing results with metabolic therapy and immunotherapy, which assist the traditional orthodox methods. I have been very blessed while researching these therapies and impressed with our outstanding success rate, as illustrated by Carolyn Gross's experience.

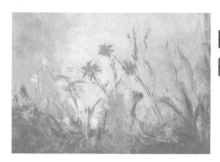

Recommended Resources

Body Care

BATHING WITH DEAD SEA SALTS

Masada Dead Sea salts can be found at health food stores like Whole Foods Market. You can also visit their website to learn more: www.masada-spa.com. These Dead Sea mineral salts are 100% natural, imported in unprocessed form from the southernmost part of the Dead Sea, where mineral concentration is the richest. The combination of these essential minerals—calcium, magnesium, and potassium—does amazing things for both mind and body. Here are some of the benefits listed:

- Soothes itching, burning, and bites
- Smoothes and softens skin
- Encourages skin to renew itself
- Helps scars to heal
- Relieves tired, aching feet and leg muscles
- Eases tension in hands and wrists

DEAD SEA SALTS IN BULK

There is a website, www.scasalt.com, that offers bulk Dead Sea salts in 5 lb.–50 lb. bags. The packaging is mylar bags, so you have to be cautious to seal them up after each use to preserve freshness. For serious bathers on a budget, this is a great resource.

ORGANIC DEODORANTS

A California-based company called Erbaviva specializes in luxury body care products. It makes a fabulous organic deodorant that comes in two fragrances: Lemon & Sage and Jasmine & Grapefruit. This upscale deodorant offers a healthy alternative for people looking to avoid aluminum, an irritant that may be absorbed in the body, used in antiperspirants. This product works to combat odor. When I wear it, I get compliments on my "perfume"! Visit www.erbaviva.com to purchase or call (877) 372-2848.

Another company, Weleda, makes a high-end organic deodorant with a Sage Rosemary fragrance and Jasmine as well. This European line is high end and available at Whole Foods Market and upscale health food stores. Visit www.weleda.com.

DETOXIFYING FOOT BATHS

When I was first diagnosed, my lower legs were sore and stiff from the accumulation of toxins that my body had acquired from the cancer. Toxins naturally accumulate around the ankles and feet because gravity pulls them there. Now there is an effective method to relieve this soreness and release toxins naturally that is being offered by spas, chiropractors, and healing centers. Detoxifying foot baths providing a low electrical current that stimulates the body to detoxify it are a very effective way to release these toxins. The treatment lasts thirty minutes, but the effect on the body lasts forty-eight hours. You need to drink trace minerals and/or electrolytes during the bath, so you don't get lightheaded, especially if you are diabetic. Visit www.AquaDetoxUSA.com or call (704) 662-9239 to find a location near you.

Mineral Salts

My *five-star suggestion* when it comes to detoxifying salts is a product from *Anakiri* called Andean Mineral Salts. They come from volcanic soils and have a high mineral content that makes them worth the investment; they are superb.

They also carry Bioenergetic Skin Care and have a Nourish Moisture Gel that stimulates the immune system. There is something unique about these products, and the bioenergetic title is accurate. Visit www.anakiri.com to order this fine line.

Books

- *An Alternative Medicine Definitive Guide to Cancer*, W. John Diamond, M.D., and Lee Cowden, M.D. This is a one thousand plus page textbook; you can purchase by calling American Metabolic Institute-Hospital San Martin (619) 267-1007 or www.amazon.com.

- *Alternative in Cancer Therapy: The Complete Guide to Non-traditional Treatments*, Ross Pelton, R.Ph., Ph.D. and Lee Overholser, Ph.D.

- *Beating Cancer with Nutrition*, Patrick Quillin, Ph.D., R.D., CNS— a comprehensive book on food supplements and nutritional strategies.

- *Elephants in Your Tent*: *Spiritual Support as a Mystic Survives Cancer*, Judith Larkin Reno, Ph.D. Available from www.amazon.com or www.treatableandbeatable.com.

- *Healing Springs: The Ultimate Guide to Taking the Waters*, Nathaniel Altman. This book will get you in the mood to visit healing mineral waters. The author provides detailed information about the health benefits of mineral water and has listed over three hundred sites for readers to indulge in.

- *Staying Healthy with the Seasons* and *The Detox Diet*, Dr. Elson Haas. The first title is a good reference for getting the benefits of specific foods and detoxification rituals during each of the four seasons. *The Detox Diet* is his latest endeavor.

- *You Can Heal Your Life*, Louise Hays. This book contains plenty of positive affirmations and thoughts for emotional healing from her years of battling cancer.

- *Outsmart Your Cancer: Alternative Non-Toxic Treatments That Work*, Tanya Harter Pierce. This book details alternative cancer treatments that are available now.

Detoxification Programs

SPAS PROGRAMS

When you are through with treatment, another way to reward your-self and improve your health is to do a detoxification week at a spa or health center once a year. At these establishments, expect fresh-made juice, fasting, detoxification rituals, and exercise. Here are some well-known spas that offer detoxification programs: Red Mountain Spa, Utah, Lake Austin Spa in Austin, Texas, The Regency House in Hallandale Florida, and the New Age Health Spa in Neversink, New York.

MEDICALLY-SUPERVISED PROGRAMS

You don't have to be a cancer patient to experience Dr. Rubio's work. At the American Metabolic Institute-Hospital San Martin (call 619-267-1107), he offers detoxification programs that are medically supervised. If you have a medical history or any medical concerns, I'd recommend doing your detoxification with a skilled medical team, at least the first time. This is also a fabulous gift to give a cancer survivor to help him or her get ready for a new approach to life.

Healing Retreats and Resources

HEALING ART

Santa Fe, New Mexico, Pippin Meikle Fine Art Gallery. Aleta Pip-pins' art helped keep my spirits lifted during months of treatment and renewal time at home. Her image was used for this book cover. Aleta has a gallery in Santa Fe, New Mexico; if you're in the area, don't miss this place. Pippin Meikle Fine Art, 236 Delgado Street, Santa Fe, New Mexico 87501; phone (505) 992-0400 or visit the gallery's website: www.pippinmeiklefineart.com.

HEALING JOURNALS

Treatable and Beatable Companion Journal by Carolyn Gross. All the suggested journaling exercises for a *treatable and beatable mindset* are contained in this companion journal to make the process of cancer recovery life enriching. Inspirational quotes and healing reminders make this a special place for cancer patients to visit with their pens. To purchase the companion journal, call toll free (866) 246-0462 or visit www.treatableandbeatable.com.

Some of my favorite journals for years have come from Brush Dance. They offer a variety of colorful and thoughtful journals; check out their website, www.brushdance.com.

MINERAL HOT SPRINGS

Healing waters that come from deep within the earth are a treat for maximizing healing and the power of rejuvenating waters. It's like nature's best kept secret, the restorative experience these waters provide. Most locations provide mineral pools for the experience called "taking of the waters." To find locations near you, search the Internet for "mineral springs" and enter your state or city. See what you come up with.

SPA RESOURCE

The Spa Connection—if you want to partake in all these wonderful spa retreats and detoxification programs and don't know where to start, here is the expert to ensure a successful experience. Contact The Spa Connection at (303) 756-9939 and ask for Lori Feiner Goldberg. She offers discounts and knows all the details on spas worldwide and will make your renewal time the best. Visit the Spa Connection's website at www.spaconnection.com.

SPA RETREATS

Throughout the year, Carolyn does spa retreats on *Women's Wellness* and *Managing Chaos with Confidence*. These events are held at some of the most prestigious spas in the country. Visit www.creativelife solutions.com/events.php or call toll free (866) 246-0462 for more information.

SWIMMING WITH THE DOLPHINS

If you are a good swimmer, love the ocean, and are ready to accelerate your healing, give yourself this gift of swimming with the dolphins. This takes place in Kona on the Big Island of Hawaii. Captains Mike and Melainah Yee are great people who have a passion for their work. Just a trip to their website will make you feel better (www.sunlightonwater.com) or call (808) 896-2480 to get more information and make this dream come true.

TREATABLE AND BEATABLE CANCER EVENTS

Visit our website for the nationwide list of Treatable and Beatable Cancer Retreats. If you'd like to sponsor one in your area, contact us toll free (866) 246-0462; we will provide you with the event information packet. All weekend retreats and one-day programs are designed to teach patients how to claim their power and get the latest treatment options for all phases of self-care, during and after treatment. These concepts reinforce the *treatable and beatable mindset* by promoting greater self-awareness and supporting individuals in finding their new approach to life. Visit www.treatableandbeatable.com.

Supplements

Protective Breast Formula by Enzematic Therapy—this superior natural product has vitamin D, calcium, tumeric rhizome extract, grape seed extract, Maitake mushroom extract, green tea leaf extract and more. Call (866) 796-3517 or visit www.protectivebreast.com; this product is also available at health food stores like Whole Foods Market.

Vaccine Trials

Studies using vaccines are listed on the National Cancer Institute website: www.cancer.gov (click on "Clinical Trials"). Last time I visited this website there was a trial for breast cancer patients to receive immunotherapy after surgery. Regionally, there are also specific trials, like this site for patients in the San Francisco Bay Area: www.breast cancertrials.org. I cannot vouch for any of these sites or trials, but I want you to find what is best for you.

Recommended Websites

- American Metabolic Institute www.amihealth.com
- National Cancer Institute www.cancer.gov
- *New England Journal of Medicine*: www.nejm.org
- Northern Inyo Hospital: www.nih.org
- Cancer Forums: www.cancerforums.net
- All About Cancer: www.cancer.org
- Nevada Cancer Institute: www.nevadacanccrinstitute.org
- The Wellness Community: www.thewellnesscommunity.org

GIVE THE GIFT OF

TREATABLE AND BEATABLE
Healing Cancer Without Surgery
TO YOUR FRIENDS AND COLLEAGUES

CHECK YOUR LEADING BOOKSTORE OR ORDER HERE

❑ **YES**, I want _____ copies of *Treatable and Beatable* at $19.95 each, plus $4.95 shipping per book (California residents please add $1.55 sales tax per book). Canadian orders must be accompanied by a postal money order in U.S. funds. Allow 15 days for delivery.

❑ **YES**, I would also like to order _____ copies of Carolyn Gross's *Staying Calm in the Midst of Chaos* at $14.95 each, plus $4.95 shipping per book (California residents please add $1.16 sales tax per book). Canadian orders must be accompanied by a postal money order in U.S. funds. Allow 15 days for delivery.

❑ **YES**, I am interested in having Carolyn Gross speak or give a seminar to my company, association, school, or organization. Please send information.

My check or money order for $_____ is enclosed.

Please charge my: ❑ Visa   ❑ MasterCard
                   ❑ Discover   ❑ American Express

Name _____

Organization _____

Address _____

City/State/Zip _____

Phone_____   Email _____

Card # _____

Exp. Date_____ Signature _____

Please make your check payable and return to:
Creative Living Publications
306 NW El Norte Parkway #426 • Escondido, CA 92026

Call your credit card order to: (866) 246-0462
www.treatableandbeatable.com   www.creativelifesolutions.com